Fuel For Life

Fuel For Life

Nutritional Wisdom

Sam Loray

Mohammed Altaf Hussain

CONTENTS

INDEX

Chapter 1: Introduction to Nutritional Wisdom

Chapter 2: The Foundations of Nutritional Wisdom

Chapter 3: The Gut-Brain Connection

Chapter 4: Superfoods and Nutrient-Rich Choices

Chapter 5: Navigating Dietary Trends

Chapter 6: Mindful Eating Practices

6.1 Introducing the concept of mindful eating and its impact on overall health.

6.2 Techniques for cultivating awareness during meals to enhance digestion and promote better food choices.

6.3 Mindful eating exercises and practices.

Chapter 7: Personalized Nutrition

7.1 Exploring the idea that there is no one-size-fits-all approach to nutrition.

7.2 Discussing genetic factors, individual differences.

7.3 The importance of adapting dietary choices to personal needs and preferences.

Chapter 8: Overcoming Challenges and Barriers

8.1 Addressing common obstacles to maintaining a healthy diet.

8.2 Strategies for overcoming emotional eating, time constraints, and other challenges.

8.3 Tips for building a supportive environment for nutritional success.

Chapter 9: Sustaining Nutritional Wisdom for a Lifetime

9.1 Summarizing key takeaways from the book.

9.2 Providing a roadmap for integrating nutritional wisdom into a long-term, sustainable lifestyle.

9.3 Encouraging ongoing learning and adaptation as nutritional science evolves.

Chapter 1

Introduction to Nutritional Wisdom

Nourishing insight is a multi-layered idea that incorporates the mind boggling connection between human wellbeing and the food we eat. It goes past simple dietary decisions and dives into the significant comprehension of how supplements, bioactive mixtures, and dietary examples impact our prosperity at the sub-atomic, cell, and fundamental levels. This acquaintance points with disentangle the layers of dietary insight, investigating its authentic roots, logical establishments, and useful ramifications for encouraging ideal wellbeing.

Authentic Points of view:

The investigation of dietary insight returns us to antiquated human advancements, where the association among food and wellbeing was profoundly imbued in social practices and philosophical convictions. Antiquated Greek logicians, for example, Hippocrates underlined the meaning of diet in keeping up with wellbeing and forestalling sickness, authoring the renowned expression, "Let food be thy endlessly medication be thy food." Correspondingly, conventional Chinese medication and Ayurveda in India perceived the mending properties of explicit food varieties and the significance of adjusting energies inside the body.

Since the beginning of time, various societies created special dietary customs in view of nearby assets, environment, and wellbeing needs. These customs frequently contained intrinsic insight went down through ages, adding to the variety of dietary practices around the world. Notwithstanding, with the coming of industrialization and globalization, customary dietary insight has confronted difficulties, prompting a shift towards handled and comfort food varieties.

Logical Establishments:

In the twentieth 100 years, logical headways pushed the comprehension of nourishment from a plainly visible to a minute level. The distinguishing proof of fundamental supplements and the explanation of their jobs in biochemical cycles denoted a change in outlook in wholesome science. The revelation of nutrients, minerals, and macronutrients laid the preparation for understanding the many-sided trap of connections that oversee human wellbeing.

The field of nutrigenomics arose, disentangling the exchange among hereditary qualities and sustenance. It uncovered that people might answer distinctively to similar dietary intercessions in view of their hereditary cosmetics.

This customized way to deal with sustenance accentuated the requirement for custom-made dietary suggestions, perceiving the uniqueness of every individual's hereditary profile.

The microbiome, an immense environment of microorganisms living in the stomach, arose as a vital participant in nourishing wellbeing. Research enlightened the advantageous connection between the microbiome and the human host, impacting digestion, safe capability, and, surprisingly, mental wellbeing. Dietary decisions were found to shape the piece of the microbiome, highlighting the significance of a reasonable and various eating routine for generally prosperity.

The Intricacy of Present day Diets:

While logical advancement gave important bits of knowledge, the healthful scene turned out to be progressively complicated in the cutting edge time. The overflow of handled food sources, high in refined sugars, undesirable fats, and counterfeit added substances, presented new difficulties to general wellbeing. Inactive ways of life and the ascent of ongoing sicknesses powered by unfortunate dietary decisions provoked a reassessment of nourishing rules.

Wholesome insight in the contemporary setting includes exploring through clashing data and knowing the genuine effect of dietary decisions on wellbeing. The ascent of nourishment deception on the web, combined with advertising procedures advancing trend abstains from food, added layers of disarray for people looking for direction on good dieting. In the midst of this intricacy, the significance of decisive reasoning and proof based direction became central.

Healthful Insight By and by:

Applying healthful insight to day to day existence requires an all encompassing methodology that goes past calorie counting and macronutrient proportions. It includes developing care around food decisions, taking into account the nature of supplements, and grasping the social and ecological ramifications of dietary propensities.

Entire, natural food varieties become the dominant focal point in a healthfully shrewd eating routine. Organic products, vegetables, entire grains, lean proteins, and sound fats give a different exhibit of supplements fundamental for physiological capabilities. Taking on a "food as medication" outlook lines up with the old insight of utilizing diet to advance wellbeing and forestall sickness.

The idea of careful eating urges people to enjoy each nibble, pay attention to craving and completion signs, and value the tactile parts of dinners. This training encourages a better relationship with food, tending to close to home and constant eating designs that might add to overconsumption and poor healthful decisions.

Social and territorial dietary examples offer significant experiences into nourishing insight. The Mediterranean eating regimen, for instance, known for its accentuation on olive oil, fish, and plant-based food varieties, has been related with various medical advantages, including cardiovascular wellbeing and life span. Understanding and integrating such dietary examples can give an outline to building healthfully sound and socially important dinners.

Difficulties and Potential open doors:

Regardless of the abundance of information accessible, a few difficulties continue advancing nourishing insight on a worldwide scale. Financial variables, food uncertainty, and differences in admittance to nutritious food sources make obstructions to taking on smart dieting propensities. Furthermore, clashing dietary suggestions from different sources add to disarray, making it moving for people to pursue informed decisions.

Tending to these difficulties requires a multi-layered approach that includes policymakers, medical services experts, instructors, and the food business. Drives pointed toward further developing food proficiency, advancing reasonable farming practices, and making evenhanded admittance to nutritious food varieties can add to a better and more educated society.

Innovation presents the two difficulties and open doors chasing after dietary insight. While falsehood multiplies on advanced stages, creative devices and applications can engage people to go with informed dietary decisions. From customized nourishment applications in light of hereditary information to stages that associate buyers with nearby, manageable food sources, innovation can possibly reshape the manner in which we approach sustenance.

Past Individual Wellbeing:

Dietary insight stretches out past individual wellbeing to envelop more extensive natural and cultural aspects. Our decisions with respect to food creation, appropriation, and utilization have expansive ramifications for the planet. Maintainable and regenerative rural works on, diminishing food waste, and supporting neighborhood food frameworks are vital parts of a healthfully shrewd methodology that thinks about the interconnectedness of human and natural wellbeing.

Worldwide issues, for example, environmental change and biodiversity misfortune highlight the criticalness of taking on dietary examples that limit natural effect. Plant-based eats less, for example, definitely stand out enough to be noticed for their capability to diminish ozone depleting substance discharges and save normal assets. Coordinating biological contemplations into wholesome insight lines up with the idea of "planetary wellbeing," underlining the relationship of human and natural prosperity.

1.1 Overview of the importance of nutrition for a healthy and fulfilling life.

The significance of nourishment in cultivating a sound and satisfying life couldn't possibly be more significant. Nourishment fills in as a basic point of support for generally speaking prosperity, impacting physical, mental, and close to home well-being. From the earliest phases of life to the brilliant years, the effect of dietary decisions resounds through each part of human life. This outline dives into the diverse meaning of sustenance, looking at its part in development and advancement, illness avoidance, mental capability, profound prosperity, and life span.

Development and Advancement:

Nourishment assumes an essential part in the development and improvement of people, especially during basic stages like outset, youth, and puberty. Satisfactory admission of fundamental supplements is basic for the development of tissues, organs, and bones. During outset, bosom milk or equation gives the essential supplements to ideal development, supporting the improvement of the mind, invulnerable framework, and other indispensable frameworks.

Youth and immaturity address times of quick development and development, requiring expanded energy and supplement admission. Supplements like calcium, vitamin D, and protein are significant for bone turn of events, guaranteeing the fulfillment of pinnacle bone mass, which is a determinant of skeletal wellbeing over the course of life. Deficient nourishment during these early stages can prompt hindered development, formative postponements, and a compromised starting point for future wellbeing.

Sickness Anticipation and The board:

Sustenance is an integral asset in the counteraction and the executives of different illnesses and ailments. A decent and supplement thick eating regimen adds to the support of a solid body weight, decreasing the gamble of stoutness and related conditions like sort 2 diabetes, cardiovascular illnesses, and certain tumors. The connection between dietary decisions and ongoing sicknesses highlights the preventive capability of embracing a wellbeing cognizant way to deal with nourishment.

Explicit supplements likewise assume key parts in illness anticipation. Cancer prevention agents, found in leafy foods, assist with killing destructive free revolutionaries, shielding cells from oxidative harm and diminishing the gamble of ongoing sicknesses. Omega-3 unsaturated fats, plentiful in greasy fish and flaxseeds, have been related with cardiovascular wellbeing and the counteraction of provocative circumstances.

In situations where people as of now face wellbeing challenges, nourishment turns into a significant part of the board and recuperation.

Clinical nourishment treatment, custom-made dietary intercessions recommended by medical care experts, is used to address conditions like diabetes, hypertension, and gastrointestinal problems. The restorative capability of sustenance stretches out past drug intercessions, featuring the significance of food as a principal part of medical care.

Mental Capability and Emotional well-being:

The multifaceted connection among sustenance and mental capability is progressively perceived, with proof recommending that dietary examples can influence mind wellbeing and mental prosperity. Omega-3 unsaturated fats, for instance, are fundamental to the construction of synapse films and have been related with mental capability and state of mind guideline. The Mediterranean eating regimen, wealthy in organic products, vegetables, entire grains, and solid fats, has been connected to a lower hazard of mental degradation and neurodegenerative illnesses.

Micronutrients like nutrients B6, B12, and folate assume fundamental parts in synapse union, adding to mental cycles and close to home dependability. Lacks in these nutrients have been embroiled in conditions like sorrow and mental disabilities. The stomach cerebrum hub, a bidirectional correspondence framework between the stomach and the mind, further stresses the impact of nourishment on emotional well-being. The stomach microbiome, molded by dietary decisions, has been connected to mind-set, stress reaction, and mental capability.

In the domain of psychological well-being, sustenance is arising as a modifiable variable that can supplement conventional mediations. The field of wholesome psychiatry investigates the associations among diet and psychological wellness, recommending that specific dietary examples might impact the gamble of mental issues. As the comprehension of these associations develops, integrating wholesome techniques into emotional well-being care might offer new roads for avoidance and treatment.

Close to home Prosperity and Personal satisfaction:

Past its physiological effects, sustenance essentially impacts close to home prosperity and generally speaking personal satisfaction. The connection among food and temperament is perplexing, including both organic and psychosocial factors. Certain food sources, like those wealthy in starches, can impact the creation of serotonin, a synapse related with state of mind guideline. Nonetheless, the effect of nourishment on temperament stretches out past individual supplements to incorporate dietary examples and way of life factors.

Slims down high in handled food sources, added sugars, and unfortunate fats have been connected to an expanded gamble of sadness and uneasiness. Conversely, counts calories stressing entire food sources, like the Mediterranean or Run (Dietary Ways to deal with Stop Hypertension) consumes less calories, have been related with better psychological well-being results. The job of nourishment in profound prosperity features the significance of taking on a comprehensive way to deal with wellbeing that coordinates physical and mental aspects.

Hydration, frequently ignored in conversations of sustenance, is a key part of prosperity. Parchedness can impede mental capability, temperament, and actual execution. Satisfactory water admission is fundamental for keeping up with cell capabilities, controlling internal heat level, and supporting supplement transport. Incorporating careful hydration rehearses into day to day existence adds to generally imperativeness and mental sharpness.

Life span and Maturing:

Nourishment assumes a urgent part in the maturing system and the mission for a long and sound life. As people age, their wholesome requirements might change, requiring changes in dietary examples to address explicit wellbeing concerns. The protection of bulk, bone thickness, and mental capability becomes vital in advancing a top notch of life during the maturing system.

Calcium and vitamin D, for instance, keep on being fundamental for bone wellbeing in more established grown-ups to forestall osteoporosis and cracks. Satisfactory protein consumption becomes critical for keeping up with bulk and capability, supporting in general portability and autonomy. Cancer prevention agent rich food varieties add to cell wellbeing and may relieve the effect of oxidative pressure related with maturing.

The job of sustenance in life span reaches out past forestalling age-related sicknesses to affecting the maturing system at the phone level. Caloric limitation, without unhealthiness, has been read up for its capability to broaden life expectancy and improve healthspan — the time of life spent healthy. While the common sense of supported caloric limitation is discussed, the investigation of supplement rich, calorie-thick weight control plans as a way to help solid maturing is a functioning area of exploration.

Functional Contemplations for a Sound Eating routine:

Accomplishing the full range of advantages presented by nourishment requires reasonable contemplations and a decent way to deal with dietary decisions. A sound eating regimen envelops different supplement thick food sources from all nutrition types, stressing the accompanying key parts:

Products of the soil: These are rich wellsprings of nutrients, minerals, fiber, and cancer prevention agents. Mean to remember a bright exhibit of products of the soil for your day to day feasts to guarantee a different scope of supplements.

Entire Grains: Pick entire grains over refined grains to profit from the additional fiber, nutrients, and minerals. Quinoa, earthy colored rice, oats, and entire wheat are great decisions.

Protein Sources: Incorporate an assortment of protein sources in your eating routine, like lean meats, poultry, fish, vegetables, nuts, and seeds. Protein is fundamental for muscle upkeep, safe capability, and by and large cell wellbeing.

Sound Fats: Consolidate wellsprings of solid fats, like avocados, olive oil, nuts, and greasy fish, into your eating regimen. These fats support mind wellbeing, chemical creation, and the assimilation of fat-solvent nutrients.

Dairy or Dairy Options: Guarantee a satisfactory admission of calcium and vitamin D for bone wellbeing. Pick low-fat or sans fat choices in the event that you consume dairy items.

Hydration: Drink a lot of water over the course of the day to keep up with ideal hydration. Limit the utilization of sweet drinks and unnecessary caffeine, as they can add to parchedness.

Limit Handled Food sources and Added Sugars: Limit the admission of handled food varieties, sweet bites, and refreshments high in added sugars. These add to abundance calorie utilization and may miss the mark on supplements.

Balance and Piece Control: Practice control in your food decisions and focus on segment sizes. Careful eating, which includes relishing each chomp and paying attention to yearning and completion signs, can add to better dietary patterns.

1.2 The impact of food choices on physical and mental well-being.

The effect of food decisions on physical and mental prosperity is significant and broad, impacting each part of a singular's life. From the cell level to the intricacies of the brain, the supplements got from the food varieties we devour assume a urgent part in forming our general wellbeing. This investigation digs into the perplexing associations between food decisions and physical and mental prosperity, looking at the systems by which nourishment impacts the body and psyche.

Actual Prosperity:

Cell Capability and Energy Digestion:

At the most central level, food fills in as the fuel that drives the cell hardware of the body. The macronutrients — sugars, proteins, and fats — got from food are separated into atoms that give energy to cell capabilities. Adenosine triphosphate (ATP), the energy money of cells, is created through cycles like glycolysis, the citrus extract cycle, and oxidative phosphorylation, all of which rely upon the accessibility of supplements.

Starches, as glucose, are an essential energy hotspot for cells, especially the mind. Proteins, made out of amino acids, assume fundamental parts in building and fixing tissues, while fats, as well as giving energy, are essential to cell layer structure and the union of chemicals. The complicated equilibrium of these macronutrients is urgent for supporting cell capability and in general energy digestion.

Body Sythesis and Weight The executives:

Past cell capability, food decisions altogether impact body structure and weight the board. The, not set in stone by the connection between energy admission and consumption, is a critical consider keeping a solid weight. Consuming a bigger number of calories than the body needs prompts weight gain, while a calorie deficiency brings about weight reduction.

The sorts of food varieties picked add to this situation. Entire, supplement thick food sources give fundamental nutrients, minerals, and fiber while offering satiety, which manages hunger and forestall gorging. Interestingly, exceptionally handled and energy-thick food sources frequently need dietary benefit, prompting abundance calorie utilization and adding to weight gain.

An eating regimen wealthy in natural products, vegetables, entire grains, and lean proteins upholds a sound body structure by giving fundamental supplements and advancing a harmony between energy admission and use. Conversely, eats less high in refined sugars, unfortunate fats, and handled food varieties are related with weight and related medical problems, including metabolic disorder and cardiovascular illnesses.

Cardiovascular Wellbeing:

The effect of food decisions reaches out to cardiovascular wellbeing, impacting risk factors, for example, pulse, cholesterol levels, and aggravation. Slims down high in immersed and trans fats, ordinarily tracked down in handled and broiled food sources, add to raised degrees of low-thickness lipoprotein (LDL) cholesterol, expanding the gamble of atherosclerosis and coronary illness.

On the other hand, consolidating unsaturated fats, like those tracked down in olive oil, avocados, and greasy fish, has been related with worked on cardiovascular results. Omega-3 unsaturated fats, specifically, tracked down in overflow in fish, flaxseeds, and pecans, have mitigating properties and add to heart wellbeing by diminishing blood thickening and further developing lipid profiles.

The job of dietary fiber in cardiovascular wellbeing is important. Dissolvable fiber, present in natural products, vegetables, and entire grains, helps lower cholesterol levels and direct glucose. Moreover, an eating regimen wealthy in potassium, tracked down in organic products, vegetables, and vegetables, adds to circulatory strain guideline, further supporting cardiovascular prosperity.

Bone Wellbeing:

Nourishment assumes a basic part in keeping up with bone wellbeing and forestalling conditions like osteoporosis. Calcium, phosphorus, magnesium, and vitamin D are key supplements engaged with bone arrangement and mineralization. Dairy items, verdant green vegetables, nuts, and sustained food sources are superb wellsprings of these supplements.

Satisfactory calcium consumption, especially during pre-adulthood and youthful adulthood, is vital for accomplishing top bone mass, which fills in as a defensive variable against bone misfortune further down the road. Vitamin D, acquired through daylight openness and dietary sources, works with the retention of calcium and adds to bone wellbeing. Keeping an eating regimen wealthy in these supplements, combined with weight-bearing activity, is fundamental for forestalling bone-related problems and breaks.

Mental Prosperity:

Synapses and Mind Capability:

The effect of food decisions on mental prosperity is progressively perceived, with proof recommending that particular supplements impact synapse union and mind capability. Synapses, the synthetic couriers of the cerebrum, assume a urgent part in managing state of mind, perception, and conduct.

Tryptophan, an amino corrosive tracked down in protein-rich food varieties, is a forerunner to serotonin, a synapse related with state of mind guideline. Starches work with the passage of tryptophan into the mind, adding to the union of serotonin and advancing a feeling of prosperity. The perplexing exchange between dietary proteins and carbs highlights the significance of adjusted feasts in supporting psychological wellness.

Omega-3 unsaturated fats, tracked down in greasy fish, flaxseeds, and pecans, are basic to the construction of cell layers in the cerebrum and have been related with mental capability and mind-set guideline. Lacks in omega-3 unsaturated fats have been connected to an expanded gamble of state of mind problems and mental degradation.

Stomach Mind Pivot:

The stomach mind pivot, a bidirectional correspondence framework between the stomach and the cerebrum, further underscores the association among sustenance and mental prosperity. The stomach microbiome, a different local area of micro-organisms dwelling in the gastrointestinal system, assumes an essential part in this correspondence organization.

Dietary decisions altogether influence the structure of the stomach microbiome. Consumes less calories high in fiber, prebiotics, and matured food sources support the development of valuable microorganisms, advancing a solid stomach climate. The aging of dietary filaments by these microorganisms delivers short-chain unsaturated fats, which have been embroiled in mind capability and emotional well-being.

Arising research recommends that lopsided characteristics in the stomach micro-biome, known as dysbiosis, may add to conditions like discouragement and nervous-ness. Probiotics, valuable microbes tracked down in matured food varieties and enhancements, have shown guarantee in tweaking the stomach cerebrum pivot and impacting mental prosperity.

Aggravation and Psychological well-being:

Ongoing aggravation, frequently connected with unfortunate dietary decisions, has been connected to emotional well-being problems. Slims down high in handled food sources, sugars, and undesirable fats add to fundamental aggravation, which might affect the mind and compound circumstances like gloom and nervousness.

On the other hand, calming eats less carbs wealthy in organic products, vegetables, entire grains, and omega-3 unsaturated fats might have defensive impacts against emo-tional wellness issues. The Mediterranean eating routine, described by its accentuation on these calming food varieties, has been related with a lower hazard of melancholy.

Glucose Guideline:

The guideline of glucose levels is urgent for supported energy and mental capabil-ity. Slims down high in refined starches and sugars lead to fast spikes and crashes in glucose, adding to exhaustion, peevishness, and trouble concentrating.

Offsetting dinners with a blend of complicated starches, proteins, and sound fats directs glucose levels, giving a consistent arrival of energy to help mental lucidity and concentration. Also, fiber-rich food sources slow the assimilation of glucose, adding to stable glucose levels and supported energy over the course of the day.

Incorporating Physical and Mental Prosperity:

Perceiving the interconnectedness of physical and mental prosperity highlights the significance of a coordinated way to deal with nourishment. Instead of survey actual wellbeing and psychological well-being as discrete areas, understanding how they commonly impact each other empowers people to settle on comprehensive decisions that advance by and large prosperity.

Careful Eating:

Careful eating is a training that urges people to be available and mindful during feasts, cultivating a more profound association with the tangible experience of eating. This approach stresses paying attention to yearning and completion prompts, enjoying flavors and surfaces, and developing a non-critical consciousness of food decisions.

By integrating care into dietary patterns, people can foster a better relationship with food, tending to profound and ongoing eating designs that might influence both physical and mental prosperity. Careful eating advances a feeling of fulfillment and delight from dinners, adding to a good and adjusted way to deal with sustenance.

Comprehensive Way of life Decisions:

Active work, sufficient rest, and stress the executives are fundamental parts of an all encompassing way to deal with prosperity.

These way of life factors cross with sustenance to make an exhaustive starting point for wellbeing. Ordinary activity upholds metabolic wellbeing, improves temperament through the arrival of endorphins, and supplements the physiological advantages got from nutritious food decisions.

Quality rest is fundamental for mental capability, temperament guideline, and generally speaking prosperity. Unfortunate rest examples and disturbances in circadian rhythms might impact dietary inclinations and lead to sub-par food decisions. Focusing on satisfactory and relaxing rest adds to mental flexibility and supports sound healthful propensities.

1.3 Introduction to the concept of nutritional wisdom and its role in making informed dietary decisions.

The idea of wholesome insight exemplifies a comprehensive and informed way to deal with pursuing dietary choices that decidedly influence by and large wellbeing and prosperity. It goes past the shortsighted perspective on food as simple food, diving into the multifaceted connection between sustenance, way of life, and individual wellbeing. In this presentation, we investigate the embodiment of healthful insight, its verifiable roots, logical establishments, and pragmatic applications in exploring the mind boggling scene of dietary decisions.

Grasping Wholesome Insight:

At its center, healthful insight includes the capacity to arrive at cognizant and informed conclusions about food, taking into account the dietary substance as well as the more extensive setting of individual requirements, social impacts, and natural manageability. It incorporates a profound comprehension of how dietary decisions impact actual wellbeing, mental prosperity, and the interconnectedness of human and planetary wellbeing.

Healthful insight recognizes the variety of human bodies and perceives that one-size-fits-all dietary suggestions may not be appropriate for everybody. It stresses a customized way to deal with nourishment, considering variables, for example, hereditary qualities, age, orientation, action level, and wellbeing status. Thusly, healthful insight engages people to pursue decisions that line up with their one of a kind necessities and add to their general essentialness.

Authentic Roots:

The underlying foundations of dietary insight can be followed back to old human advancements, where the natural association among food and wellbeing was profoundly imbued in social practices and philosophical convictions. Old Greek rationalists, including Hippocrates, underlined the significance of diet in keeping up with wellbeing, begetting the notable expression, "Let food be thy endlessly medication be thy food." This point of view laid the basis for the comprehension that food could assume a part in fulfilling hunger as well as in advancing prosperity and forestalling sickness.

Likewise, customary Chinese medication and Ayurveda in India perceived the recuperating properties of explicit food varieties and the significance of adjusting energies inside the body. These old frameworks of medication saw food as a wellspring of sustenance as well as for the purpose of fitting the body, psyche, and soul. The insight implanted in these verifiable points of view established the groundwork for a comprehensive comprehension of nourishment that rises above the reductionist methodology predominant in present day times.

Logical Establishments:

The twentieth century denoted a critical jump in the logical comprehension of sustenance, moving from fundamental ideas of fundamental supplements to a more nuanced investigation of the perplexing connections among diet and wellbeing. The disclosure of nutrients, minerals, and macronutrients gave a system to figuring out the particular jobs of individual supplements in supporting physiological capabilities.

The development of nutrigenomics, a field that inspects the cooperation among hereditary qualities and sustenance, added a layer of intricacy to the comprehension of dietary effect on wellbeing. Nutrigenomics uncovered that people might answer distinctively to similar food sources in light of their hereditary cosmetics, featuring the requirement for customized dietary proposals.

The microbiome, a huge local area of microorganisms dwelling in the stomach, turned into a point of convergence in wholesome exploration. The microbiome's job in processing, supplement retention, and resistant capability highlighted the harmonious connection between the microbial world and human wellbeing. Dietary decisions were found to shape the structure of the microbiome, impacting its variety and usefulness.

The Intricacy of Present day Diets:

In the contemporary scene, the idea of wholesome insight faces difficulties in the midst of the wealth of handled and comfort food sources. The shift towards industrialized food creation, combined with stationary ways of life, has added to an ascent in diet-related persistent illnesses. The commonness of profoundly handled food varieties, wealthy in refined sugars, unfortunate fats, and fake added substances, has prompted worries about the nourishing nature of current eating regimens.

In exploring this intricacy, people are besieged with clashing data about what comprises a sound eating regimen. Craze eats less carbs, frequently advanced without hearty logical proof, gain prevalence, adding disarray to the journey for ideal nourishment. The pervasiveness of nourishment falsehood on the web further entangles the scene, making it moving for people to observe solid counsel from pseudoscience.

Healthful Insight By and by:

Applying dietary insight practically speaking includes a diverse methodology that stretches out past calorie counting and macronutrient proportions. It requires a cognizant and careful commitment with food decisions, taking into account the nature of supplements, the social setting of eating, and the ecological effect of dietary choices.

Entire, Natural Food varieties: At the center of nourishing insight is the accentuation on eating entire, natural food varieties. Organic products, vegetables, entire grains, lean proteins, and sound fats give a rich exhibit of fundamental supplements without the added substances and additives frequently tracked down in handled food sources.

Social and Territorial Contemplations: Nourishing insight perceives the variety of dietary examples across societies and areas. Customary weight control plans, molded by nearby assets and social practices, frequently offer significant bits of knowledge into adjusted and wellbeing advancing dietary patterns. Understanding and integrating these social subtleties into dietary decisions add to both nourishing and social prosperity.

Careful Eating: The act of careful eating includes being available and completely connected with during dinners. It incorporates relishing each nibble, focusing on craving and totality signals, and valuing the tangible parts of food. Careful eating cultivates a better relationship with food, advancing a cognizant and purposeful way to deal with sustenance.

Customized Nourishment: Dietary insight recognizes the independence of healthful requirements. Customized sustenance, informed by variables like hereditary qualities and wellbeing status, perceives that what works for one individual may not work for another. Fitting dietary decisions to individual prerequisites upgrades the viability of healthful intercessions and supports long haul prosperity.

Difficulties and Valuable open doors:

In spite of the natural worth of wholesome insight, a few difficulties hinder its boundless reception. Financial elements, remembering differences for admittance to new and nutritious food varieties, add to disparities in dietary propensities. Tending to these inconsistencies requires an exhaustive methodology that consolidates instructive drives, strategy changes, and local area based mediations.

The ascent of sustenance deception represents a critical test to healthful insight. Unconfirmed cases and trend diets can lead people down ways that may not line up with their wellbeing objectives. Advancing media proficiency and decisive reasoning abilities is fundamental to engage people to observe proof based data from sensationalized or deluding content.

Innovation, while adding to the scattering of sustenance data, likewise presents open doors for advancing wholesome insight. Portable applications, online stages, and advanced assets can give open and customized data, assisting people with pursuing informed dietary decisions. Coordinating innovation into nourishment training and emotionally supportive networks improves the span and effect of wholesome insight drives.

Past Individual Wellbeing:
Nourishing insight stretches out past individual wellbeing to envelop more extensive cultural and natural aspects. Individuals decisions with respect to food creation, appropriation, and utilization have significant ramifications for the planet. Manageable and moral contemplations become basic parts of dietary insight as people perceive their job in supporting a strong and regenerative food framework.

Manageable Horticulture: Dietary insight lines up with the standards of maintainable agribusiness, stressing rehearses that advance soil wellbeing, biodiversity, and water protection. Supporting neighborhood and regenerative cultivating rehearses adds to the natural manageability of food creation.

Lessening Food Squander: A healthfully savvy approach includes limiting food squander. Being aware of part measures, using extras innovatively, and supporting drives that address food squander add to reasonable utilization designs.

Plant-Based Diets: Plant-based slims down, wealthy in natural products, vegetables, vegetables, and entire grains, certainly stand out for their capability to lessen the ecological effect of food creation. Wholesome insight perceives the advantages of integrating plant-based decisions into dietary examples to help both individual wellbeing and ecological maintainability.

Support for Food Equity: Wholesome insight stretches out to upholding for food equity — an idea that underscores evenhanded admittance to nutritious food varieties for all. Resolving fundamental issues of food instability and advancing strategies that improve admittance to new and reasonable food varieties are indispensable parts of a socially mindful way to deal with sustenance.

The idea of nourishing insight assumes a critical part in directing people towards settling on educated and careful dietary choices. It fills in as a compass in the complicated scene of sustenance, offering a comprehensive methodology that stretches out past shortsighted ideas of consuming less calories and calorie counting. In this investigation, we dive into the multi-layered job of nourishing insight in molding dietary choices, grasping its effect on individual wellbeing, and perceiving its more extensive ramifications for cultural and ecological prosperity.

All encompassing Comprehension of Nourishment:

Healthful insight welcomes people to move past a reductionist perspective on nourishment that centers exclusively around the detached parts of food — calories, macronutrients, and micronutrients. All things considered, it energizes a comprehensive comprehension that considers the interconnectedness of different variables impacting dietary decisions.

At its center, wholesome insight perceives that food isn't simply a wellspring of fuel however an intricate framework of mixtures that interface with the human body at numerous levels. It recognizes the synergistic impacts of supplements, the significance of entire food sources, and the job of dietary examples in molding in general wellbeing. This all encompassing point of view engages people to see the value in the significant effect of their dietary decisions on physical, mental, and profound prosperity.

Informed Independent direction:

One of the basic parts of dietary insight is the accentuation on informed navigation. This includes developing a basic outlook, looking for solid data, and knowing proof based suggestions from prevailing fashions and deception. In the time of data overburden, where nourishment patterns and diets multiply via web-based entertainment and the web, wholesome insight turns into a device for exploring the clamor and pursuing decisions grounded in science and individual necessities.

Informed independent direction additionally includes grasping individual healthful necessities. Nourishing insight perceives that people have novel hereditary cosmetics, medical issue, and way of life factors that impact their wholesome requirements. Fitting dietary decisions to line up with these singular elements guarantees that wholesome objectives are sensible, feasible, and steady of long haul prosperity.

Verifiable Roots and Social Contemplations:

To grasp the profundity of healthful insight, investigating its verifiable roots and the impact of social contemplations on dietary decisions is important. Authentic viewpoints on food and wellbeing, as found in antiquated customs and methods of reasoning, add to the primary standards of nourishing insight.

Old Greek scholars, for example, Hippocrates, laid the foundation for the comprehension that food has restorative properties. Customary Chinese medication and Ayurveda perceived the job of adjusted sustenance as one inside the body. These authentic experiences illuminate nourishing insight by accentuating the interconnectedness of food, wellbeing, and prosperity.

Social contemplations further advance healthful insight by recognizing the variety of dietary examples across various social orders. What comprises a sound eating regimen might differ in view of social standards, local accessibility of food sources, and culinary practices.

Nourishing insight urges people to appreciate and coordinate these social subtleties into their dietary decisions, encouraging a feeling of association with legacy and advancing variety in food utilization.

Logical Establishments and Nutrigenomics:

The logical groundworks of dietary insight lie in the headways made in nourishing science, especially in understanding how supplements connect with the body at a sub-atomic level. The ID of fundamental supplements, the revelation of nutrients and minerals, and the clarification of their jobs in physiological cycles add to the logical premise of dietary insight.

Nutrigenomics, a field that investigates the connection among hereditary qualities and sustenance, adds a layer of intricacy to healthful comprehension. It uncovers that people might answer contrastingly to similar food varieties in view of their hereditary cosmetics. Wholesome insight consolidates this customized viewpoint, perceiving that there is nobody size-fits-all way to deal with diet and that individualized sustenance can enhance wellbeing results.

Useful Utilizations of Wholesome Insight:

Entire, Natural Food sources: A foundation of dietary insight is the accentuation on entire, natural food sources. These food sources, like organic products, vegetables, entire grains, lean proteins, and sound fats, give a range of supplements in their normal structures. Wholesome insight urges people to focus on these food varieties over handled and refined choices, perceiving their unrivaled nourishing substance and wellbeing advancing properties.

Careful Eating: The act of careful eating is a pragmatic utilization of dietary insight. Careful eating includes being available during dinners, relishing each chomp, and focusing on appetite and completion prompts. By developing mindfulness and care around dietary patterns, people can encourage a better relationship with food, forestall indulging, and get more prominent fulfillment from their dinners.

Social Joining: Healthful insight perceives the significance of social combination in dietary decisions. It urges people to investigate and embrace the assorted culinary customs that line up with their social foundations. This upgrades the tactile delight in feasts as well as guarantees that dietary decisions are socially significant, encouraging a feeling of association and character.

Customized Sustenance: Understanding and applying healthful insight includes fitting dietary decisions to individual necessities. Customized nourishment considers factors like age, orientation, wellbeing status, and hereditary inclinations. This customized approach guarantees that dietary proposals are sensible, reachable, and steady of individual wellbeing objectives.

Decisive Reasoning and Media Proficiency: In the period of data, wholesome insight involves the advancement of decisive reasoning abilities and media education.

It includes fundamentally assessing nourishment data, recognizing tenable sources from deception, and pursuing decisions in view of proof as opposed to patterns. By improving these abilities, people can explore the frequently befuddling scene of sustenance guidance and pursue choices that line up with their wellbeing targets.

Difficulties and Open doors:

While wholesome insight offers a structure for going with informed dietary choices, it faces moves that should be tended to for broad reception. Financial elements, remembering incongruities for admittance to new and nutritious food varieties, present difficulties to carrying out nourishing insight for an expansive scope. Tending to these variations requires deliberate endeavors in schooling, strategy changes, and local area based drives to guarantee that everybody has the potential chance to settle on good food decisions.

Nourishment falsehood is one more critical test to dietary insight. Unverified cases, craze counts calories, and pseudoscientific counsel can lead people down ways that may not line up with their wellbeing objectives. Advancing media proficiency, training on decisive reasoning, and clear correspondence of proof based nourishment data are fundamental parts of conquering this test.

Mechanical progressions present the two difficulties and potential open doors for dietary insight. While the web and advanced stages add to the dispersal of nourishment data, they likewise intensify the spread of deception. Utilizing innovation for positive results, for example, creating proof based sustenance applications, online assets, and instructive stages, can upgrade the openness of nourishing insight.

Past Individual Wellbeing:

Nourishing insight reaches out past individual wellbeing to include more extensive cultural and ecological aspects. Perceiving the interconnectedness of human and planetary wellbeing, healthful insight urges decisions that add to the prosperity of both.

Reasonable and Moral Contemplations: Nourishing insight lines up with practical and moral contemplations in food decisions. It includes supporting cultivating rehearses that focus on soil wellbeing, biodiversity, and water protection. Picking morally obtained and reasonably delivered food sources turns into a fundamental part of nourishing insight, recognizing the effect of dietary choices on the soundness of the planet.

Diminishing Food Squander: Dietary insight remembers a concentration for lessening food squander. Being aware of piece sizes, using extras innovatively, and supporting drives that address food squander add to reasonable utilization designs. This lines up with ecological maintainability as well as advances mindful and cognizant food utilization.

Plant-Based Diets for Ecological Maintainability: Recognizing the natural effect of food decisions, healthful insight might include contemplations of plant-based slims down. Plant-based eats less, wealthy in organic products, vegetables, vegetables, and entire grains, are related with lower ecological impressions. Picking plant-based choices turns into a cognizant choice to help both individual wellbeing and the supportability of the planet.

Support for Food Equity: Nourishing insight stretches out to promotion for food equity — a methodology that accentuates impartial admittance to nutritious food sources for all. Resolving fundamental issues of food frailty, supporting local area drives, and advancing strategies that improve admittance to new and reasonable food varieties become vital parts of a socially dependable way to deal with sustenance.

Chapter 2

The Foundations of Nutritional Wisdom

Nourishment is a complex field that interlaces science, culture, and individual decisions. The groundworks of nourishing insight are based upon an intricate snare of elements, incorporating natural necessities, social impacts, and the powerful exchange between individual wellbeing and more extensive cultural settings. To genuinely comprehend the substance of nourishing insight, one should dig into the mind boggling balance between logical information and the different woven artwork of human ways of life.

At the center of dietary insight lies the central comprehension of the human body's wholesome prerequisites. The mind boggling dance of macronutrients — sugars, proteins, and fats — and micronutrients — nutrients and minerals — shapes the groundwork of a solid eating regimen. These fundamental supplements assume vital parts in different physiological cycles, from energy creation to resistant capability. Perceiving the multifaceted requirements of the body is the most important move towards developing nourishing insight.

Starches, frequently considered the body's essential energy source, come in different structures — straightforward sugars and complex carbs. The utilization of entire grains, organic products, and vegetables gives a consistent arrival of energy, cultivating supported essentialness. Proteins, made out of amino acids, are the structure blocks of tissues, muscles, and compounds. A different protein consumption, got from both creature and plant sources, guarantees the body's primary respectability and supports crucial biochemical responses.

Fats, long attacked, are urgent for cell structure, chemical creation, and supplement retention. The harmony among soaked and unsaturated fats, alongside a familiarity with trans fats, highlights the nuanced understanding expected for nourishing insight. It isn't only about the amount yet in addition the nature of fats consumed, underscoring sources like avocados, nuts, and olive oil.

In the domain of micronutrients, nutrients and minerals go about as impetuses for biochemical responses, managing physiological cycles with accuracy. The rainbow of leafy foods, each offering a special exhibit of nutrients and minerals, delineates the significance of dietary variety. Calcium, magnesium, potassium, L-ascorbic acid, and incalculable others add to the unpredictable orchestra that supports life.

Be that as it may, wholesome insight rises above the simple specification of supplements. It reaches out into the social aspects that shape our dietary decisions. Culture fills in as a powerful force to be reckoned with, deciding what we eat as well as how we see food. Customary cooking styles, went down through ages, epitomize food as well as a rich embroidery of legacy, ceremonies, and social bonds.

Investigating social subtleties divulges the insight implanted in conventional weight control plans. The Mediterranean eating regimen, commended for its heart-sound advantages, represents the joining of supplement rich food sources with social practices. Olive oil, plentiful in monounsaturated fats, turns out to be in excess of a culinary fixing — it represents a lifestyle. Essentially, the Japanese hug of fish and matured food varieties reflects an amicable relationship with nature and a promise to wellbeing.

However, social impacts are not restricted to geological limits. In the cutting edge period, globalization has introduced a combination of culinary practices, making a different and interconnected gastronomic scene. The ascent of combination food reflects the developing idea of dietary decisions, as individuals draw motivation from different societies to make extraordinary, customized ways to deal with sustenance.

Additionally, the social setting encompassing food can't be ignored. Eating rises above simple food; a public demonstration ties people and networks together. The common experience of a dinner cultivates social union, supporting the social and close to home components of sustenance. Understanding healthful insight involves perceiving the collective parts of food, recognizing its job in festivals, ceremonies, and familial bonds.

In any case, the social setting additionally presents difficulties. The pervasiveness of inexpensive food, stationary ways of life, and the rushed speed of present day life have modified customary examples of eating. The comfort of handled food varieties frequently comes at the expense of healthy benefit, prompting an incomprehensible situation where overflow coincides with hunger. Wholesome insight, in this way, requires a basic assessment of cultural designs and a cognizant work to explore the cutting edge food scene.

Chasing wholesome insight, the idea of careful eating arises as a core value. Careful eating rises above the simple demonstration of utilization; it includes a significant familiarity with the tangible experience, the affirmation of craving and satiety signals, and a cognizant association with the starting points of the food. Developing care in dietary patterns encourages a more significant relationship with food, enabling people to pursue informed decisions lined up with their wellbeing objectives.

Also, the harmonious connection among sustenance and mental prosperity high-lights the all encompassing nature of dietary insight.

Arising research enlightens the complex associations among diet and psychological wellness, featuring the effect of supplements on mind-set, perception, and generally mental flexibility. The stomach mind pivot, a bidirectional correspondence frame-work between the stomach and the cerebrum, underscores the interconnectedness of physical and psychological well-being.

The reconciliation of wholesome insight into psychological well-being care pro-claims a change in perspective, perceiving the job of nourishment as a modifiable figure mental prosperity. Consumes less calories wealthy in omega-3 unsaturated fats, cancer prevention agents, and entire food sources exhibit likely advantages in over-seeing conditions like despondency and tension. As the logical comprehension of this perplexing relationship extends, dietary intercessions might become indispensable parts of emotional well-being treatment systems.

Moreover, the ecological aspect can't be separated from the groundworks of dietary insight. Our decisions with respect to food creation, circulation, and utilization have significant ramifications for the planet. Manageable practices, like natural cultivating, moral obtaining, and diminishing food squander, line up with the standards of wholesome insight by perceiving the interconnectedness of human wellbeing and the soundness of the planet.

The natural impression of our dietary decisions reaches out past the plate. The industrialization of farming, the overreliance on monocultures, and the unnecessary utilization of pesticides add to natural debasement. The shift towards regenerative farming, agroecological practices, and plant-based slims down mirrors an aggregate acknowledgment of the requirement for naturally cognizant food frameworks.

Fundamentally, wholesome insight includes an agreeable incorporation of individual wellbeing, social mindfulness, social elements, mental prosperity, and ecological manageability. It rises above reductionist methodologies that emphasis exclusively on detached supplements, pushing for an all encompassing comprehension of food as a multi-layered substance that sustains the body, psyche, and planet.

The excursion towards nourishing insight is a unique interaction, requiring non-stop learning, transformation, and an eagerness to embrace different viewpoints. It requests a takeoff from prescriptive dietary doctrines and urges people to pay atten-tion to their bodies, perceiving the exceptional beneficial interaction between private prosperity and more extensive biological contemplations.

Instructive drives assume a crucial part in dispersing wholesome insight to different networks. Engaging people with the information and abilities to pursue informed dietary decisions encourages a feeling of organization and independence. Sustenance training goes past the scattering of realities; it develops decisive reasoning, empowering people to explore the intricate scene of healthful data with wisdom.

Also, overcoming any barrier between logical exploration and public comprehension is central. The interpretation of logical discoveries into available, proof based rules engages people to settle on decisions lined up with their wellbeing objectives. Clear correspondence channels between researchers, wellbeing experts, and the overall population are fundamental to neutralize falsehood and advance a nuanced comprehension of sustenance.

The job of policymakers in molding the dietary scene couldn't possibly be more significant. Authoritative measures that elevate admittance to nutritious food varieties, control food publicizing, and boost manageable farming practices add to the formation of a climate helpful for dietary insight. The incorporation of nourishing proficiency into school educational programs guarantees that people in the future are furnished with the information and abilities to settle on informed dietary decisions.

All in all, the underpinnings of wholesome insight rest upon a multi-faceted structure that embraces the perplexing exchange between organic, social, social, mental, and ecological variables. An excursion rises above the simple demonstration of eating, developing into a significant comprehension of the harmonious connection between private wellbeing and the prosperity of the planet. Healthful insight isn't an objective however a consistent, powerful cycle — an investigation of the significant associations that tight spot us to the food we eat and the world we possess.

2.1 Exploring the basics of macronutrients and micronutrients.

Understanding the complexities of sustenance requires digging into the primary components that comprise our dietary admission: macronutrients and micronutrients. These fundamental parts structure the structure blocks of an even eating routine, assuming unmistakable parts in keeping up with ideal wellbeing and supporting different physiological capabilities.

Macronutrients, as the name recommends, are supplements that the body expects in moderately huge amounts. They envelop starches, proteins, and fats, each contributing interestingly to the body's energy needs and by and large prosperity. Carbs, found in food sources like grains, organic products, and vegetables, act as the essential wellspring of energy for the body. They are separated into glucose, giving fuel to different cell exercises and supporting physical processes.

Proteins, involved amino acids, are critical for the arrangement and fix of tissues, compounds, and chemicals. Meat, dairy items, vegetables, and nuts are rich wellsprings of protein, guaranteeing that the body has the essential unrefined components for keeping up with primary respectability and working with fundamental biochemical cycles. The variety of amino acids in various protein sources highlights the significance of integrating an assortment of protein-rich food sources into one's eating routine.

Fats, frequently misconstrued and unjustifiably trashed, are essential to by and large wellbeing. They are fundamental for cell film structure, chemical creation, and the ingestion of fat-solvent nutrients (A, D, E, and K). Solid fats, like those tracked down in avocados, nuts, seeds, and olive oil, add to cardiovascular wellbeing and backing different physical processes. Finding some kind of harmony between various sorts of fats — immersed, unsaturated, and polyunsaturated — is critical to streamlining the advantages of fat admission.

In opposition to macronutrients, micronutrients are expected in more modest amounts however are similarly fundamental for keeping up with wellbeing. Micronutrients envelop nutrients and minerals, each assuming explicit parts in different physiological cycles. Nutrients are natural mixtures that help development, improvement, and by and large prosperity. They can be water-solvent (e.g., L-ascorbic acid, B nutrients) or fat-solvent (e.g., vitamin A, D, E, K), and their presence in a reasonable eating routine is urgent for forestalling inadequacies and supporting ideal wellbeing.

Minerals, then again, are inorganic components important for a scope of physiological capabilities, including bone wellbeing, nerve capability, and liquid equilibrium. Calcium, for example, is essential for bone strength and muscle capability, while iron is urgent for oxygen transport in the blood. Consolidating a different cluster of organic products, vegetables, entire grains, and incline proteins toward one's eating routine guarantees a sufficient stock of these micronutrients.

The exchange among macronutrients and micronutrients makes a sensitive equilibrium that supports the body's mind boggling capabilities. For instance, the retention of non-heme iron (found in plant-based food varieties) is upgraded within the sight of L-ascorbic acid, exhibiting the synergistic connection between various supplements. This interconnectedness stresses the significance of eating different food sources to meet the body's assorted dietary requirements.

While the comprehension of macronutrients and micronutrients is fundamental, the idea of bioavailability adds one more layer of intricacy. Bioavailability alludes to the degree to which the body can ingest and use supplements from a given food source. Factors, for example, cooking techniques, food handling, and the presence of different mixtures in the eating regimen can impact the bioavailability of supplements.

Cooking, for example, can upgrade the bioavailability of specific supplements while reducing others. Intensity can separate the cell walls of plants, making supplements more available. Then again, a few nutrients, similar to L-ascorbic acid, are delicate to warm and can be lost during cooking. The decision of cooking techniques, consequently, turns into an essential thought in safeguarding the dietary substance of food sources.

Food handling likewise assumes a part in supplement bioavailability. Profoundly handled food varieties frequently go through adjustments that can strip them of fundamental supplements. Refining grains, for instance, eliminates the wheat and microbe, diminishing the fiber and supplement content. Interestingly, entire grains hold their regular structure, giving a more extravagant wellspring of supplements.

The presence of specific mixtures in food sources can either improve or hinder supplement assimilation. For example, oxalates and phytates, normally happening intensifies in some plant food sources, can tie to minerals like calcium and iron, lessening their assimilation. Nonetheless, the synchronous utilization of L-ascorbic acid rich food sources can balance this impact, featuring the significance of dietary variety and cooperative energy in supplement assimilation.

Wholesome necessities shift across people in light of elements, for example, age, sex, action level, and wellbeing status. Fitting dietary decisions to meet explicit necessities is fundamental for advancing in general prosperity. For example, competitors might have higher energy and protein prerequisites to help their preparation, while pregnant ladies need expanded folic corrosive and iron to help fetal turn of events.

Exceptional consideration should likewise be given to populaces with extraordinary healthful requirements, like babies and the old. Bosom milk, frequently thought to be the highest quality level for baby nourishment, gives an equilibrium of macronutrients and micronutrients vital for development and improvement. As people age, supplement ingestion might diminish, accentuating the requirement for supplement thick food varieties to meet fundamental necessities.

Dietary examples and inclinations further add to the individualization of wholesome requirements. Social and strict practices, moral contemplations, and individual decisions shape dietary propensities, affecting the sorts and amounts of food sources devoured. Veggie lover and vegetarian eats less carbs, for instance, discard specific creature items, requiring cautious intending to guarantee satisfactory admission of fundamental supplements like B12, iron, and omega-3 unsaturated fats.

The idea of dietary quality reaches out past the simple arrangement of fundamental supplements. It embraces the more extensive setting of food decisions, accentuating the significance of entire, negligibly handled food sources in advancing wellbeing. Entire food sources, in their regular state, offer a range of supplements and phytochemicals that add to in general prosperity.

Conversely, the over the top utilization of super handled food sources, loaded down with added substances, additives, and refined sugars, has been related with different medical problems.

These food varieties frequently give void calories, coming up short on the healthful thickness tracked down in entire food varieties. The shift towards focusing on entire, supplement thick food sources lines up with the standards of advancing macronutrient and micronutrient sufficiency as well as by and large dietary quality.

General wellbeing suggestions, directed by broad exploration, give a system to accomplishing ideal dietary status. Dietary rules, frequently gave by wellbeing specialists, frame general suggestions for the utilization of various nutrition types to address healthful issues and diminish the gamble of constant sicknesses. These rules act as important devices for people and medical care experts in advancing wellbeing through informed dietary decisions.

Nonetheless, the execution of dietary rules faces difficulties on different fronts. Financial variables, social variety, and individual inclinations add to fluctuated adherence to these proposals. Admittance to new, supplement thick food sources might be restricted in specific networks, prompting abberations in nourishing admission. Also, clashing data in the media and the pervasiveness of craze diets can make disarray, impeding the reception of proof based dietary practices.

The acknowledgment of the powerful idea of nourishment, impacted by developing logical comprehension and cultural changes, requires a persistent reexamination of dietary suggestions. Research on the stomach microbiome, customized sustenance, and the effect of food creation on the climate adds to a more nuanced comprehension of dietary examples and their suggestions for wellbeing.

The arising field of nourishing genomics, or nutrigenomics, investigates the cooperation between qualities, diet, and wellbeing. It dives into how individual hereditary varieties impact reactions to dietary parts, preparing for customized sustenance suggestions. The acknowledgment that hereditary variables assume a part in supplement digestion adds one more layer of intricacy to the generally complex trap of nourishing science.

As we explore the intricacies of nourishment, perceiving the job of conduct factors in forming dietary choices is fundamental. Dietary patterns are impacted by physiological appetite as well as by profound, ecological, and expressive gestures. Careful eating, a methodology that supports an increased consciousness of the eating experience, advances a better relationship with food and can add to worked on dietary decisions.

The socio-social parts of food utilization likewise assume a huge part in forming dietary ways of behaving. Food is frequently interlaced with social customs, festivities, and close to home encounters. The demonstration of sharing a dinner cultivates social bonds, and social practices around food add to a feeling of personality and having a place. Recognizing the social elements of sustenance highlights the requirement for socially delicate ways to deal with dietary direction.

Simultaneously, the predominance of food showcasing, particularly for profoundly handled and energy-thick items, represents a test to smart dieting ways of behaving. The universality of promoting, combined with the openness of comfort food varieties, adds to the worldwide ascent in non-transferable sicknesses. Tending to these difficulties requires a diverse methodology that includes people as well as policymakers, the food business, and the health.

2.2 Understanding the body's energy needs and the role of carbohydrates, proteins, and fats.

To understand the complicated interchange of sustenance inside the human body, it is basic to unwind the secrets encompassing energy needs and the jobs played by macronutrients — explicitly, carbs, proteins, and fats. These macronutrients act as the establishment for supporting life, supporting fundamental physiological capabilities, and giving the energy expected to day to day exercises.

Starches, frequently situated as a key member in the energy game, are the body's liked and essential wellspring of fuel. Found in different food varieties like grains, natural products, vegetables, and vegetables, carbs are made out of sugars, starches, and filaments. Upon utilization, these mixtures go through processing, at last separating into glucose — a straightforward sugar that fills in as the body's essential energy cash.

Understanding the body's energy needs includes perceiving the mind boggling course of glucose digestion. Once ingested into the circulatory system, glucose is moved to cells all through the body, where it goes through glycolysis — a progression of enzymatic responses that convert glucose into ATP (adenosine triphosphate), the cell energy cash. The energy delivered during this interaction powers different cell exercises, empowering capabilities going from muscle constrictions to the blend of biomolecules.

Nonetheless, the body's energy needs are not exclusively met via carbs. Proteins, made out of amino acids, likewise add to the energy pool. While proteins assume a urgent part in primary parts like muscles, tissues, and catalysts, they can be changed over into energy under particular conditions. During times of expanded energy requests or lacking starch consumption, the body might fall back on separating proteins through an interaction called gluconeogenesis to create glucose for energy.

Fats, frequently misconstrued and criticized, are one more fundamental player in the energy scene. Containing fatty substances, fats are put away in fat tissue and act as a concentrated wellspring of energy. At the point when the body requires more energy than what is promptly accessible from sugars, it takes advantage of these fat stores through lipolysis, separating fatty oils into unsaturated fats and glycerol. The unsaturated fats go through beta-oxidation, yielding ATP and satisfying the body's energy needs.

Starches, proteins, and fats on the whole add to the day to day caloric admission, estimated in kilocalories (kcal). Understanding the harmony between these macronutrients is essential for addressing energy needs while guaranteeing ideal wellbeing. The Dietary Rules for Americans suggest that starches comprise 45-65% of all out everyday calories, proteins make up 10-35%, and fats involve 20-35%.

The idea of macronutrient conveyance highlights the significance of a reasonable eating routine. Starches, with their nearby accessibility as an energy source, are especially pivotal for people taking part in proactive tasks. Perseverance competitors, for instance, frequently depend on starches to support energy levels during delayed work out. Conversely, a stationary way of life or explicit medical issue might require changes in carb admission to forestall unreasonable caloric utilization.

Proteins, past their job in energy arrangement, are fundamental to the body's design and capability. Amino acids, the structure blocks of proteins, are classified into fundamental and unnecessary. Fundamental amino acids should be gotten from the eating regimen since the body can't blend them. A shifted protein consumption from both creature and plant sources guarantees the accessibility of all fundamental amino acids, supporting ideal development, tissue fix, and chemical capability.

Fats, however thick in calories, are fundamental for various physiological cycles. The nature of fats, as opposed to sheer amount, is of central significance. Immersed fats, generally tracked down in creature items and a few tropical oils, can add to cardiovascular issues when consumed in overabundance. Then again, unsaturated fats, tracked down in olive oil, avocados, and nuts, advance heart wellbeing and add to generally prosperity.

Understanding the body's energy needs additionally includes perceiving the powerful idea of energy balance. The mind boggling interchange between energy consumption (calories consumed) and energy use (calories consumed) decides if the body keeps up with, gains, or gets in shape. Caloric overabundance prompts weight gain, while a calorie deficiency brings about weight reduction. Accomplishing an energy offset that lines up with individual objectives requires an attention to both dietary decisions and actual work levels.

The body's energy needs shift across people in view of elements, for example, age, sex, weight, movement level, and digestion. Basal metabolic rate (BMR), the energy consumed very still, represents most of everyday energy consumption. Factors impacting BMR incorporate lean weight, age, and hereditary qualities. Actual work and the thermic impact of food, addressing the energy expected for assimilation, retention, and digestion of supplements, further add to add up to energy use.

Starches assume a significant part in filling actual work. The body stores starches as glycogen in muscles and the liver. During exercise, these glycogen stores are separated to give a promptly accessible wellspring of glucose, supporting energy levels. Perseverance competitors frequently take part in carb stacking — expanding carb admission before an occasion — to boost glycogen stores and improve execution.

Proteins, past their primary job, add to muscle capability and fix, making them fundamental for people participated in obstruction preparing or those looking to assemble and keep up with bulk. The timing and dissemination of protein admission over the course of the day impact muscle protein combination. Consuming satisfactory protein post-practice works with muscle recuperation and transformation, supporting in general actual execution.

Fats, regardless of their relationship with put away energy, assume a vital part in perseverance exercises. During delayed work out, the body movements to using a higher extent of fat for energy, saving glycogen stores. This variation, known as metabolic adaptability, features the body's capacity to switch between various fuel sources in light of the power and span of actual work.

The connection among sustenance and exercise reaches out past energy needs. Hydration, electrolyte equilibrium, and supplement timing all add to improving execution and recuperation. Sufficient liquid admission is fundamental for forestalling lack of hydration, which can debilitate mental capability and actual execution. Electrolytes like sodium, potassium, and magnesium, lost through sweat during exercise, should be renewed to keep up with appropriate liquid equilibrium.

Supplement timing, the essential admission of supplements around the hour of activity, impacts execution and recuperation. Consuming a decent dinner or bite containing sugars and protein before practice gives the important fuel and supports muscle protein union. Post-practice sustenance, especially the admission of carbs and protein, works with glycogen recharging and muscle recuperation.

While understanding macronutrients is essential, the nature of the eating regimen is similarly pivotal. The accentuation on entire, insignificantly handled food varieties lines up with the standards of advancing macronutrient ampleness as well as in general dietary quality. Entire grains, organic products, vegetables, lean proteins, and solid fats give a rich exhibit of supplements, fiber, and phytochemicals that add to generally prosperity.

Alternately, the unnecessary utilization of super handled food varieties, described by elevated degrees of added sugars, sodium, and undesirable fats, presents wellbeing chances. These food varieties, frequently low in dietary benefit, add to caloric over-abundance, advance irritation, and are related with a higher gamble of persistent illnesses.

The shift towards focusing on supplement thick food sources highlights the significance of thinking about the general dietary example.

The job of carbs, proteins, and fats in the body's energy elements stretches out past the quick setting of activity and day to day exercises. The unpredictable interaction of these macronutrients adds to long haul wellbeing results and the anticipation of persistent illnesses. Awkward nature in macronutrient admission, like over the top utilization of added sugars or unfortunate fats, are connected to conditions like heftiness, diabetes, and cardiovascular illnesses.

Starches, explicitly, have been a point of convergence of conversations in regards to their effect on wellbeing. The sort and nature of carbs matter, with an accentuation on picking entire, complex starches over refined sugars. The glycemic record, a proportion of how rapidly a food raises blood glucose levels, fills in as a device for settling on informed starch decisions. Low-glycemic food varieties, which discharge glucose gradually, furnish supported energy and are related with worked on metabolic wellbeing.

Proteins, notwithstanding their job in energy arrangement, add to satiety — the sensation of completion. Remembering protein-rich food sources for dinners and bites controls hunger and may support weight the board. Also, the wellspring of protein matters; plant-based proteins, like those from vegetables, nuts, and seeds, offer extra medical advantages by giving fiber, nutrients, and minerals.

Fats, frequently examined for their caloric thickness, play a nuanced job in wellbeing. The center has moved from attacking all fats to perceiving the significance of separating between immersed, unsaturated, and trans fats. Trans fats, related with an expanded gamble of cardiovascular infections, are generally stayed away from. Unsaturated fats, found in sources like avocados, olive oil, and greasy fish, add to heart wellbeing and ought to supplant soaked fats in the eating routine.

Understanding the body's energy needs additionally requires tending to the idea of dietary examples. Diets like the Mediterranean eating regimen, portrayed by a high admission of organic products, vegetables, entire grains, and sound fats, have been related with various medical advantages. These examples, wealthy in different supplements and phytochemicals, mirror a comprehensive way to deal with nourishment that stretches out past individual macronutrients.

Nourishing science persistently advances, with continuous exploration revealing insight into the many-sided associations among diet and wellbeing. The idea of customized sustenance, recognizing individual varieties because of dietary intercessions, addresses a change in perspective. Factors, for example, hereditary qualities, stomach microbiota sythesis, and metabolic status add to the customized idea of sustenance.

As how we might interpret the body's energy needs extends, the job of macronutrients stays vital to upgrading wellbeing. Nonetheless, this understanding stretches out past simple quantitative contemplations to envelop the nature of dietary decisions, the effect on constant illnesses, and the customized idea of sustenance. Accomplishing an amicable harmony between sugars, proteins, and fats includes meeting energy prerequisites as well as cultivating in general prosperity through educated and careful dietary decisions.

2.3 Highlighting the importance of vitamins and minerals for optimal health.

The meaning of nutrients and minerals in keeping up with ideal wellbeing couldn't possibly be more significant. These micronutrients assume different and critical parts in different physiological cycles, supporting development, advancement, and the general working of the human body. Understanding their significance includes digging into the particular elements of individual nutrients and minerals and perceiving what their insufficiencies or awkward nature can mean for wellbeing.

Nutrients, named either water-solvent (e.g., L-ascorbic acid, B nutrients) or fat-dissolvable (e.g., vitamin A, D, E, K), are natural mixtures that the body expects in little amounts for fundamental capabilities. Vitamin A, for example, assumes a crucial part in vision, safe capability, and skin wellbeing. Found in food varieties like yams, carrots, and spinach, vitamin An is fundamental to keeping up with the honesty of the eyes' light-delicate cells and supporting the resistant framework.

Vitamin D, frequently alluded to as the "daylight nutrient," adds to bone wellbeing by managing calcium and phosphorus ingestion. Orchestrated in the skin in light of daylight, vitamin D is additionally tracked down in greasy fish, strengthened dairy items, and egg yolks. Its lack is related with conditions like rickets in youngsters and osteoporosis in grown-ups, underscoring the significance of sufficient vitamin D admission for skeletal wellbeing.

Vitamin E, a powerful cell reinforcement, shields cells from oxidative harm. Nuts, seeds, and vegetable oils are rich wellsprings of vitamin E, adding to the body's safeguard against free revolutionaries and supporting skin wellbeing. Vitamin K, fundamental for blood coagulating and bone digestion, is tracked down in green verdant vegetables, adding to the blend of proteins important for these critical physiological cycles.

The water-solvent nutrients, including L-ascorbic acid and the B nutrients (B1, B2, B3, B5, B6, B7, B9, B12), are engaged with a scope of capabilities. L-ascorbic acid, found in citrus organic products, strawberries, and chime peppers, is eminent for its job in collagen combination, resistant help, and cancer prevention agent action. The B nutrients, altogether known as the B-complex, take part in energy digestion, nerve capability, and DNA combination. They are plentiful in entire grains, salad greens, nuts, and vegetables.

Vitamin B12, specifically, merits consideration because of its relationship with neurological capability and red platelet creation. Found fundamentally in creature items, its lack can prompt circumstances like malevolent frailty and neurological debilitations. For people following veggie lover or vegetarian eats less, acquiring satisfactory B12 through invigorated food varieties or enhancements becomes significant for forestalling lacks.

Minerals, then again, are inorganic components that add to different physiological capabilities, going from bone wellbeing to chemical movement. Calcium, a key mineral, shapes the primary part of bones and teeth and assumes a part in muscle capability and blood thickening. Dairy items, salad greens, and braced food varieties act as great wellsprings of calcium. Its lack can bring about conditions like osteoporosis, stressing the significance of keeping up with sufficient calcium consumption over the course of life.

Magnesium, frequently alluded to as the "ace mineral," is engaged with more than 300 enzymatic responses in the body, affecting energy digestion, muscle capability, and nerve transmission. Entire grains, nuts, seeds, and mixed greens give magnesium, and its lack has been connected to conditions like muscle cramps, cardiovascular issues, and debilitated glucose digestion.

Iron, fundamental for oxygen transport in the blood, is a basic mineral, and its lack prompts frailty. While heme iron from creature sources is all the more promptly assimilated, non-heme iron from plant sources can add to generally press consumption. Matching iron-rich food sources with L-ascorbic acid rich food sources improves non-heme iron retention. Guaranteeing sufficient iron admission is especially significant for weak populaces, like pregnant ladies and people with explicit ailments.

Zinc, a minor component, upholds resistant capability, wound mending, and DNA blend. Tracked down in meat, fish, nuts, and seeds, zinc lack can think twice about resistant framework and disable development and improvement. Iodine, essential for thyroid capability and the development of thyroid chemicals, is principally acquired from iodized salt and fish. Its inadequacy can prompt thyroid brokenness and formative issues, especially during pregnancy.

Selenium, going about as a cancer prevention agent, is fundamental for safeguarding cells from oxidative harm. Fish, Brazil nuts, and entire grains are rich wellsprings of selenium. Its lack has been related with specific tumors and compromised insusceptible capability. Copper, associated with iron digestion, collagen union, and cell reinforcement guard, is tracked down in organ meats, fish, and nuts. Its lack can appear as pallor and bone anomalies.

The jobs of nutrients and minerals stretch out past individual capabilities; they frequently associate synergistically. For example, vitamin D improves calcium retention, underlining the significance of a comprehensive way to deal with supplement consumption.

Likewise, L-ascorbic acid upgrades the assimilation of non-heme iron from plant sources, exhibiting the complicated interchange among nutrients and minerals for ideal wellbeing.

Micronutrient inadequacies, while preventable, keep on being a worldwide wellbeing concern. Factors like deficient dietary admission, unfortunate food decisions, confined consumes less calories, and certain ailments add to lacks. Furthermore, financial elements, including restricted admittance to different and supplement thick food varieties, can compound the gamble of micronutrient lacks, particularly in weak populaces.

Fortress, the most common way of adding nutrients and minerals to food varieties, has been an effective methodology in tending to lacks on a populace level. Normal models incorporate the fortress of salt with iodine, milk with vitamin D, and oats with different B nutrients. Stronghold programs, when executed wisely, add to general wellbeing endeavors to ease micronutrient lacks and work on by and large prosperity.

Nonetheless, it is fundamental for work out some kind of harmony, as exorbitant admission of specific nutrients and minerals can prompt poisonousness. The "more is better" attitude doesn't turn out as expected for all micronutrients, and the idea of an Upper Admission Level (UL) is laid out to direct safe enhancement use. For instance, over the top vitamin An admission, fundamentally through supplements, can prompt poisonousness side effects like queasiness, tipsiness, and even organ harm.

The significance of nutrients and minerals goes past their old style jobs in forestalling lacks. Arising research investigates their likely in forestalling and overseeing ongoing illnesses. Cell reinforcement nutrients, like L-ascorbic acid and E, show possible advantages in decreasing oxidative pressure and aggravation, adding to cardiovascular wellbeing and relieving age-related conditions.

Vitamin D, once thought about essentially for bone wellbeing, is presently perceived for its effect on resistant capability, psychological well-being, and constant infection avoidance. Research recommends relationship between lack of vitamin D and conditions like immune system sicknesses, certain malignant growths, and temperament problems. While the causal connections are as yet being clarified, these discoveries feature the diverse jobs of nutrients in keeping up with in general wellbeing.

Additionally, minerals like zinc and selenium, known for their resistant supporting properties, are under a microscope for their true capacity in forestalling diseases and balancing provocative reactions. Satisfactory admission of these minerals is essential to supporting the body's guard components and improving wellbeing results, especially with regards to irresistible infections.

The idea of customized nourishment, taking into account individual varieties in supplement prerequisites in view of hereditary cosmetics and wellbeing status, is getting forward movement. Nutrigenomics, the investigation of how qualities impact nourishing reactions, offers experiences into how people process and use nutrients and minerals. This customized way to deal with nourishment means to fit dietary suggestions to a singular's interesting hereditary profile, improving wellbeing results.

As the logical comprehension of nutrients and minerals extends, it becomes obvious that their jobs are not segregated yet interconnected inside the more extensive setting of diet and way of life. The accentuation on entire, supplement thick food sources as wellsprings of nutrients and minerals lines up with advancing by and large dietary quality. A different and adjusted diet, wealthy in organic products, vegetables, entire grains, lean proteins, and sound fats, gives the establishment to addressing micronutrient needs and supporting ideal wellbeing.

All in all, featuring the significance of nutrients and minerals for ideal wellbeing highlights their basic jobs in different physiological capabilities. From vision and resistant help to bone wellbeing and energy digestion, these micronutrients add to the multifaceted embroidery of prosperity. As examination keeps on disentangling the intricacies of micronutrient communications and their effect on wellbeing, the accentuation on a different and adjusted diet stays a foundation of advancing by and large prosperity. Whether got through entire food sources or painstakingly chose supplements, guaranteeing sufficient admission of nutrients and minerals is a crucial part of sustaining wellbeing and imperativeness all through the life expectancy.

The basic job of nutrients and minerals in supporting ideal wellbeing is a foundation of wholesome science. These micronutrients, expected by the body in somewhat limited quantities, assume assorted and fundamental parts in physiological cycles fundamental for development, improvement, and generally prosperity. Understanding the meaning of these micronutrients includes investigating their singular capabilities, dietary sources, and the possible results of inadequacies or awkward nature.

Nutrients, ordered into water-solvent (e.g., L-ascorbic acid, B nutrients) and fat-solvent (e.g., vitamin A, D, E, K) gatherings, are natural mixtures that take part in a horde of organic capabilities. Vitamin A, for example, is significant for vision, resistant capability, and skin wellbeing. Tracked down in food sources like yams, carrots, and mixed greens, vitamin A backings the upkeep of the eyes' light-delicate cells and adds to a hearty safe framework.

Vitamin D, frequently alluded to as the "daylight nutrient," is necessary to bone wellbeing as it controls the ingestion of calcium and phosphorus. Combined in the skin upon openness to daylight, vitamin D is additionally present in greasy fish, sustained dairy items, and egg yolks. Its lack is related with conditions like rickets in kids and osteoporosis in grown-ups, highlighting the significance of adequate vitamin D admission for skeletal wellbeing.

Vitamin E, a powerful cell reinforcement, shields cells from oxidative harm. Nuts, seeds, vegetable oils, and salad greens are rich wellsprings of vitamin E, adding to the body's guard against free revolutionaries and supporting skin wellbeing. Vitamin K, imperative for blood thickening and bone digestion, is tracked down in overflow in green verdant vegetables. Sufficient vitamin K admission guarantees the combination of proteins fundamental for these basic physiological cycles.

Water-dissolvable nutrients, including L-ascorbic acid and the B nutrients (B1, B2, B3, B5, B6, B7, B9, B12), partake in many capabilities. L-ascorbic acid, plentifully present in citrus natural products, strawberries, and chime peppers, is eminent for its part in collagen amalgamation, resistant help, and cancer prevention agent action. The B nutrients all in all add to energy digestion, nerve capability, and DNA combination. They are tracked down in entire grains, mixed greens, nuts, and vegetables.

Vitamin B12 merits extraordinary consideration because of its relationship with neurological capability and red platelet creation. Fundamentally obtained from creature items, its lack can prompt circumstances like vindictive sickliness and neurological weaknesses. People following veggie lover or vegetarian slims down need to painstakingly design their admission to forestall B12 lacks through strengthened food varieties or enhancements.

Minerals, inorganic components that add to different physiological capabilities, are similarly crucial for ideal wellbeing. Calcium, a significant mineral, is critical for bone and teeth structure, muscle capability, and blood thickening. Dairy items, mixed greens, and braced food sources are superb wellsprings of calcium. Keeping up with satisfactory calcium consumption over the course of life is foremost to forestall conditions like osteoporosis.

Magnesium, frequently alluded to as the "ace mineral," partakes in more than 300 enzymatic responses, impacting energy digestion, muscle capability, and nerve transmission. Entire grains, nuts, seeds, and salad greens give magnesium, and its inadequacy is connected to issues, for example, muscle cramps, cardiovascular issues, and disabled glucose digestion.

Iron, fundamental for oxygen transport in the blood, is a basic mineral. While heme iron from creature sources is all the more promptly assimilated, non-heme iron from plant sources adds to generally press admission. Guaranteeing adequate iron admission is imperative to forestall paleness. Zinc, a minor component, upholds safe capability, wound recuperating, and DNA combination. Zinc lack can think twice about insusceptible framework and debilitate development and improvement. It is tracked down in meat, fish, nuts, and seeds.

Iodine is vital for thyroid capability and the development of thyroid chemicals. Essential sources incorporate iodized salt and fish, and its lack can prompt thyroid brokenness and formative issues, especially during pregnancy.

Selenium, going about as a cancer prevention agent, shields cells from oxidative harm and is found in fish, Brazil nuts, and entire grains. Its inadequacy has been related with specific malignant growths and compromised resistant capability.

Copper, associated with iron digestion, collagen amalgamation, and cancer prevention agent safeguard, is tracked down in organ meats, fish, and nuts. Lack can appear as pallor and bone anomalies. Every mineral, with its interesting capabilities, adds to the perplexing embroidery of physiological cycles, underlining the requirement for a different and adjusted diet to meet these micronutrient needs.

The communications among nutrients and minerals frequently rise above their singular capabilities, exhibiting a powerful transaction that adds to by and large wellbeing. For instance, vitamin D upgrades calcium retention, stressing the significance of an all encompassing way to deal with supplement consumption. Additionally, L-ascorbic acid upgrades the ingestion of non-heme iron from plant sources, delineating the multifaceted collaboration between these micronutrients for ideal wellbeing.

Micronutrient inadequacies, however preventable, stay a worldwide wellbeing concern. Factors like deficient dietary admission, unfortunate food decisions, limited counts calories, and certain ailments add to lacks. Moreover, financial elements, including restricted admittance to different and supplement thick food sources, can worsen the gamble of micronutrient lacks, particularly in weak populaces.

Fortress, the most common way of adding nutrients and minerals to food sources, has demonstrated to be an effective procedure in tending to lacks on a populace level. Models incorporate the fortress of salt with iodine, milk with vitamin D, and grains with different B nutrients. Fortress programs, when carried out prudently, add to general wellbeing endeavors to reduce micronutrient inadequacies and work on by and large prosperity.

Notwithstanding, alert is justified, as extreme admission of specific nutrients and minerals can prompt poisonousness. The idea that "more is better" doesn't turn out as expected for all micronutrients, and the idea of an Upper Admission Level (UL) is laid out to direct safe enhancement use. Unnecessary admission of vitamin A, fundamentally through supplements, can prompt poisonousness side effects like queasiness, wooziness, and even organ harm.

Past their parts in forestalling lacks, nutrients and minerals are progressively perceived for their likely in forestalling and overseeing constant illnesses. Cancer prevention agent nutrients, like L-ascorbic acid and E, show possible advantages in decreasing oxidative pressure and irritation, adding to cardiovascular wellbeing and moderating age-related conditions.

Vitamin D, once fundamentally connected with bone wellbeing, is currently perceived for its impact on invulnerable capability, emotional well-being, and constant infection anticipation. Research proposes relationship between lack of vitamin D and conditions like immune system illnesses, certain tumors, and temperament problems.

While the causal connections are as yet being clarified, these discoveries feature the multi-layered jobs of nutrients in keeping up with in general wellbeing.

Minerals like zinc and selenium, known for their resistant helping properties, are under a magnifying glass for their true capacity in forestalling diseases and regulating provocative reactions. Satisfactory admission of these minerals is fundamental to supporting the body's guard systems and enhancing wellbeing results, especially with regards to irresistible infections.

The advancing field of customized nourishment, taking into account individual varieties in supplement prerequisites in view of hereditary cosmetics and wellbeing status, is getting some forward movement. Nutrigenomics, the investigation of how qualities impact wholesome reactions, offers bits of knowledge into how people use and use nutrients and minerals. This customized way to deal with nourishment intends to fit dietary suggestions to a singular's interesting hereditary profile, advancing wellbeing results.

As the logical comprehension of nutrients and minerals extends, it becomes obvious that their jobs are interconnected inside the more extensive setting of diet and way of life. The accentuation on entire, supplement thick food varieties as wellsprings of nutrients and minerals lines up with advancing in general dietary quality. A different and adjusted diet, wealthy in natural products, vegetables, entire grains, lean proteins, and sound fats, gives the establishment to addressing micronutrient needs and supporting ideal wellbeing.

All in all, featuring the significance of nutrients and minerals for ideal wellbeing highlights their key jobs in different physiological capabilities. From vision and safe help to bone wellbeing and energy digestion, these micronutrients add to the perplexing embroidered artwork of prosperity. As examination keeps on unwinding the intricacies of micronutrient cooperations and their effect on wellbeing, the accentuation on a different and adjusted diet stays a foundation of advancing by and large prosperity. Whether got through entire food varieties or painstakingly chose supplements, guaranteeing satisfactory admission of nutrients and minerals is a crucial part of supporting wellbeing and essentialness all through the life expectancy.

Chapter 3

The Gut-Brain Connection

The stomach cerebrum association is a complicated and captivating relationship that assumes a critical part in our general wellbeing and prosperity. This perplexing transaction between the gastrointestinal framework and the mind has been the subject of broad exploration as of late, uncovering a heap of associations that go past basic processing.

At the core of the stomach mind association is the intestinal sensory system (ENS), frequently alluded to as the "second cerebrum." This complex organization of neurons is implanted in the walls of the gastrointestinal system and works freely of the focal sensory system (CNS). The ENS speaks with the mind through the vagus nerve, making a bidirectional correspondence roadway between the stomach and the cerebrum.

One of the central participants in this correspondence network is the stomach microbiota, a different local area of trillions of microorganisms that dwell in the gastro-intestinal lot. These microorganisms, including microbes, infections, parasites, and archaea, structure a perplexing biological system that significantly impacts different parts of our wellbeing, including processing, digestion, and invulnerable capability.

The stomach microbiota and the cerebrum are in consistent correspondence through a scope of flagging pathways. This correspondence happens through the arrival of synapses, chemicals, and insusceptible framework atoms that movement between the stomach and the cerebrum. Serotonin, for instance, a synapse generally connected with temperament guideline, is essentially created in the stomach. The equilibrium of synapses in the stomach can impact mind-set, nervousness, and, surprisingly, mental capability.

Besides, the stomach microbiota assumes a pivotal part in the creation of short-chain unsaturated fats (SCFAs), which have been connected to different physiological and neurological capabilities. SCFAs, for example, butyrate, acetic acid derivation, and propionate, are created by the maturation of dietary strands by stomach microorganisms. These mixtures have been displayed to make calming impacts and may add to the support of a sound stomach hindrance.

The stomach cerebrum hub likewise balances the safe reaction, with the stomach filling in as an essential site for resistant framework enactment. The nearby cooperation between the stomach and the resistant framework has suggestions for neuro-inflammation, a cycle ensnared in the improvement of neurodegenerative illnesses and mental problems.

Lopsided characteristics in the stomach microbiota, known as dysbiosis, have been related with fiery circumstances and may add to the pathogenesis of specific neurological problems.

The effect of the stomach cerebrum association stretches out past the domains of actual wellbeing and includes mental and close to home prosperity. Research has shown that disturbances in the stomach microbiota, either through diet, anti-microbials, or different elements, can impact state of mind and conduct. Conditions like crabby entrail condition (IBS), described by gastrointestinal side effects, for example, stomach torment and adjusted gut propensities, frequently coincide with mental issues like tension and misery.

Stress, a universal part of present day life, can likewise impact the stomach cerebrum association. The arrival of stress chemicals, like cortisol, can modify the organization of the stomach microbiota and upset the equilibrium of the stomach mind hub. Persistent pressure has been connected to gastrointestinal issues and may add to the advancement of mind-set problems.

Alternately, mediations pointed toward regulating the stomach microbiota, like probiotics and prebiotics, have shown guarantee in further developing emotional wellness results. Probiotics, which are live microorganisms that present medical advantages to the host, have been researched for their capability to reduce side effects of despondency and nervousness. Prebiotics, then again, are substances that advance the development and action of advantageous stomach microbes, and their utilization has been related with further developed state of mind and mental capability.

Diet, a significant determinant of stomach microbiota piece, assumes an essential part in the stomach cerebrum association. The Western eating regimen, described by elevated degrees of handled food sources and low fiber admission, has been connected to adjustments in the stomach microbiota and expanded aggravation. Going against the norm, an eating routine wealthy in natural products, vegetables, and entire grains gives fundamental supplements and fiber that help a different and solid stomach microbiota.

The effect of the stomach cerebrum association on neurological problems is an expanding area of examination. Conditions like Parkinson's illness and Alzheimer's sickness, generally saw as basically influencing the cerebrum, are presently being examined with regards to the stomach mind pivot. Arising proof proposes that adjustments of the stomach microbiota may go before the beginning of neurodegenerative illnesses, opening new roads for early finding and mediation.

In the domain of psychiatry, the stomach cerebrum association is earning respect as an expected objective for helpful mediations. The stomach microbiota has been ensnared in temperament problems, and methodologies pointed toward regulating its organization are being investigated as adjunctive medicines for conditions like discouragement and tension.

The utilization of psychobiotics, a term begat for probiotics with psychological wellness benefits, addresses a clever way to deal with emotional well-being care.

The stomach cerebrum association is additionally personally connected to the improvement of the focal sensory system during early life. The foundation of a sound stomach microbiota in early stages is critical for the development of the safe framework and the legitimate improvement of the cerebrum. Disturbances in this cycle, whether because of cesarean segment conveyance, recipe taking care of, or early openness to anti-toxins, may have long haul ramifications for neurological and psychological well-being.

Ecological variables, including openness to contaminations and poisons, can influence the stomach mind association. The stomach fills in as an essential connection point between the outside climate and the inner milieu of the body. Accordingly, natural factors that change the stomach microbiota or compromise the respectability of the stomach obstruction can impact mind capability and may add to the etiology of neurological problems.

The ramifications of the stomach cerebrum association stretch out to the field of customized medication, where individual contrasts in stomach microbiota piece might impact reactions to prescriptions. The stomach microbiota can utilize drugs, influencing their adequacy and security. Understanding the exchange between the stomach microbiota and drug digestion is fundamental for streamlining remedial results and limiting unfavorable impacts.

All in all, the stomach cerebrum association is a dynamic and unpredictable relationship that reaches out a long ways past the domains of processing. The bi-directional correspondence between the stomach and the cerebrum, intervened by the stomach microbiota, the intestinal sensory system, and different flagging atoms, has significant ramifications for our physical, mental, and close to home prosperity. As exploration in this field keeps on propelling, the potential for outfitting the stomach mind association for helpful purposes turns out to be progressively apparent, opening new roads for further developing wellbeing across the life expectancy.

3.1 Examining the intricate relationship between gut health and mental well-being.

The multifaceted connection between stomach wellbeing and mental prosperity is a subject of developing interest and exploration inside the fields of medication and neuroscience. Customarily, the stomach has been seen as a urgent framework for processing and supplement ingestion. Notwithstanding, late logical progressions have uncovered an intricate exchange between the stomach and the mind, uncovering that these two apparently unmistakable frameworks are personally associated and apply a significant effect on one another.

At the center of this association lies the intestinal sensory system (ENS), frequently alluded to as the "second mind." The ENS is a perplexing organization of neurons implanted in the walls of the gastrointestinal lot, reaching out from the throat to the rectum. This many-sided framework works freely of the focal sensory system (CNS) yet speaks with it through the vagus nerve, making a bidirectional correspondence pivot known as the stomach mind hub.

The stomach cerebrum pivot empowers consistent correspondence between the stomach and the mind, considering the coordination of different physiological cycles. One of the critical go betweens in this correspondence network is the stomach microbiota, a different local area of microorganisms living in the gastrointestinal parcel. These microorganisms, including microscopic organisms, infections, parasites, and archaea, structure a harmonious biological system with the host and assume a crucial part in keeping up with wellbeing.

The stomach microbiota impacts different parts of wellbeing, from supplement digestion to safe framework balance. Notwithstanding, its effect on mental prosperity has arisen as an especially interesting area of study. The stomach microbiota is engaged with the development of synapses and bioactive mixtures that can influence state of mind, cognizance, and conduct. Serotonin, a synapse generally connected with mind-set guideline, is prevalently delivered in the stomach, underscoring the significance of the stomach cerebrum pivot in profound prosperity.

In addition, the stomach microbiota adds to the development of short-chain unsaturated fats (SCFAs) through the maturation of dietary strands. SCFAs, for example, butyrate, acetic acid derivation, and propionate, assume a part in keeping up with stomach wellbeing and have been displayed to apply neuroprotective impacts. These mixtures can cross the blood-mind boundary, impacting cerebrum capability and possibly alleviating the gamble of neurological issues.

The stomach mind association is additionally unpredictably connected to the safe framework. The stomach fills in as an essential site for resistant framework enactment, and the equilibrium of safe reactions in the stomach is critical for in general well-being. Dysregulation of the resistant framework in the stomach can prompt ongoing irritation, which has been embroiled in the advancement of neurological and mental problems.

Stress, a pervasive part of present day life, further highlights the intricacy of the stomach mind relationship. The arrival of stress chemicals, like cortisol, can affect the stomach microbiota organization and change the penetrability of the stomach hindrance. Ongoing pressure has been related with gastrointestinal issues, like bad tempered entrail disorder (IBS), and may add to the beginning or fuel of psychological wellness conditions.

On the other hand, mediations pointed toward regulating the stomach microbiota, like probiotics and prebiotics, have shown guarantee in affecting mental prosperity. Probiotics, which are live microorganisms presenting medical advantages to the host, have been explored for their capability to lighten side effects of melancholy and uneasiness.

Prebiotics, substances that advance the development and movement of valuable stomach microorganisms, significantly affect mind-set and mental capability.

Diet, a huge figure molding the creation of the stomach microbiota, assumes a urgent part in the stomach mind association. The Western eating routine, portrayed by elevated degrees of handled food sources and low fiber consumption, has been related with a changed stomach microbiota and expanded irritation. Conversely, an eating routine wealthy in organic products, vegetables, and entire grains gives fundamental supplements and fiber that help a different and sound stomach microbiota, with likely advantages for mental prosperity.

The effect of the stomach cerebrum association reaches out past the domains of mind-set and comprehension and envelops the field of psychiatry. Arising research proposes that disturbances in the stomach microbiota may add to the pathogenesis of different psychological wellness problems, including despondency, nervousness, and schizophrenia. Understanding the job of the stomach mind hub in mental circumstances opens new roads for restorative mediations and may reform the treatment approaches for dysfunctional behaviors.

Neurological problems, generally viewed as principally influencing the mind, are currently being investigated with regards to the stomach cerebrum pivot. Conditions, for example, Parkinson's illness and Alzheimer's sickness have been connected to modifications in the stomach microbiota, proposing an expected job for the stomach in the commencement or movement of these infections. Examining the stomach mind association in neurodegenerative problems gives an all encompassing viewpoint on sickness systems and offers novel open doors for early determination and mediation.

Early valuable encounters and the advancement of the focal sensory system are likewise intently attached to the stomach mind association. The foundation of a sound stomach microbiota during early stages is basic for the development of the resistant framework and the legitimate improvement of the mind. Disturbances in this cycle, whether because of cesarean segment conveyance, recipe taking care of, or early openness to anti-microbials, may have long haul ramifications for neurological and psychological wellness.

Ecological elements, going from openness to poisons to way of life decisions, can influence the stomach mind association. The stomach goes about as an essential connection point between the outside climate and the inward milieu of the body, making it defenseless to outer impacts. Understanding what natural variables mean for the stomach cerebrum hub is fundamental for creating methodologies to moderate their effect and advance mental prosperity.

The ramifications of the stomach cerebrum association reach out to the field of customized medication, where individual varieties in stomach microbiota sythesis may impact reactions to meds. The stomach microbiota assumes a part in drug digestion, influencing the viability and security of drug mediations.

Perceiving the effect of the stomach cerebrum pivot on drug reactions is urgent for fitting clinical medicines to individual patients and improving helpful results.

All in all, the perplexing connection between stomach wellbeing and mental prosperity is a diverse and dynamic transaction that rises above conventional limits between substantial frameworks. The stomach cerebrum hub, interceded by the intestinal sensory system, the stomach microbiota, and different flagging atoms, impacts state of mind, discernment, and conduct. As examination in this field progresses, the potential for bridling the stomach cerebrum association for helpful purposes turns out to be progressively clear, making ready for imaginative ways to deal with advance emotional well-being and prosperity.

3.2 Discussing the impact of a balanced diet on cognitive function and emotional stability.

The effect of diet on mental capability and profound security is a subject of expanding significance in the fields of sustenance, brain science, and neuroscience. The food we eat fills in as the fuel for our bodies, affecting actual wellbeing as well as the perplexing cycles of the cerebrum. As exploration propels, it turns out to be progressively obvious that a decent eating routine assumes a vital part in supporting ideal mental capability and close to home prosperity.

A fair eating regimen is portrayed by the admission of various supplements in fitting extents. This incorporates macronutrients like sugars, proteins, and fats, as well as micronutrients can imagine nutrients and minerals. Every one of these parts assumes a special part in keeping up with the soundness of the cerebrum and supporting the multifaceted cycles engaged with cognizance and close to home guideline.

Sugars, frequently defamed in specific dietary patterns, are an essential wellspring of energy for the cerebrum. Glucose, got from the breakdown of carbs, is the cerebrum's favored fuel. Consuming complex carbs, like entire grains, organic products, and vegetables, gives a supported arrival of glucose, offering a consistent stockpile of energy for mental cycles. Basic carbs, tracked down in handled food sources and sweet tidbits, may prompt fast spikes and crashes in glucose levels, possibly affecting mental capability.

Proteins are fundamental for the blend of synapses, the substance couriers that work with correspondence between synapses. Amino acids, the structure blocks of proteins, assume a pivotal part in the creation of synapses like serotonin, dopamine, and norepinephrine. Counting an assortment of protein sources in the eating routine, like lean meats, fish, dairy, vegetables, and nuts, guarantees a satisfactory stockpile of these amino acids, supporting synapse balance and mental capability.

Fats, frequently isolated into immersed and unsaturated classes, are fundamental to cerebrum wellbeing. The cerebrum is made out of a lot of fat, and dietary fats add to the underlying trustworthiness of cell layers.

Omega-3 unsaturated fats, tracked down in greasy fish, flaxseeds, and pecans, are especially significant for cerebrum capability. These unsaturated fats have been related with mental advantages and may assume a part in moderating the gamble of neuro-degenerative issues.

Micronutrients, including nutrients and minerals, are fundamental for different biochemical cycles in the cerebrum. B-nutrients, like B6, B9 (folate), and B12, are engaged with the combination of synapses and the guideline of homocysteine, a compound connected to mental degradation. Sufficient admission of nutrients like C and E, as well as minerals can imagine zinc and magnesium, adds to cell reinforcement protection and supports in general mind wellbeing.

Cell reinforcements, tracked down in overflow in products of the soil, safeguard the mind from oxidative pressure. Oxidative pressure, coming about because of an ir-regularity between free revolutionaries and cell reinforcements, has been embroiled in neurodegenerative illnesses and mental deterioration. Remembering different bright products of the soil for the eating regimen gives a range of cell reinforcements, possibly lessening the gamble old enough related mental disability.

The stomach cerebrum association, a bidirectional correspondence hub between the stomach and the mind, likewise assumes a part in mental capability and close to home strength. A reasonable eating regimen that supports stomach wellbeing, including fiber-rich food sources and probiotics, can decidedly impact the stomach microbiota. The stomach microbiota, thus, produces synapses and speaks with the cerebrum through the stomach mind hub, affecting temperament and mental cycles.

The Mediterranean eating regimen, described by an overflow of organic products, vegetables, entire grains, fish, and olive oil, has acquired consideration for its expected mental advantages. Studies have proposed that adherence to the Mediterranean eating routine is related with a decreased gamble of mental deterioration and neurodegen-erative sicknesses. The mix of supplement rich food varieties in this diet gives a comprehensive way to deal with supporting mind wellbeing.

Hydration is one more basic part of keeping up with mental capability. Drying out can hinder mental execution, consideration, and temperament. Satisfactory water admission is vital for the legitimate working of synapses and the disposal of side-effects from the mind. It is crucial for stay very much hydrated to help ideal mental and close to home prosperity.

The effect of diet on profound security is complicatedly connected to the idea of wholesome psychiatry, a field that investigates the connection among diet and emo-tional wellness. The stomach cerebrum hub, as referenced prior, assumes a critical part in this association. The stomach microbiota impacts the development of synapses like serotonin, which significantly affects mind-set guideline.

Certain dietary examples, like those high in handled food sources, sugar, and immersed fats, have been related with an expanded gamble of temperament issues, including despondency and tension. Going against the norm, consumes less calories wealthy in entire food sources, omega-3 unsaturated fats, and cell reinforcements have shown guarantee in supporting profound prosperity. The effect of nourishment on psychological well-being isn't just significant for the counteraction of issues yet additionally as a likely remedial methodology in the treatment of mind-set problems.

The impact of diet on mental capability and close to home steadiness reaches out across the life expectancy, from early improvement to maturing. During youth, appropriate nourishment is significant for mental health and mental capability. Supplement lacks during this basic period can significantly affect mental capacities and may add to learning and social issues.

In youthfulness, a period set apart by quick physical and close to home changes, healthful necessities stay critical for mental health and mental prosperity. Sufficient admission of supplements like iron, zinc, and omega-3 unsaturated fats upholds mental capability and may have suggestions for profound strength during this period of life.

In adulthood, the requests on mental capability proceed, and the effect of diet on mental deterioration turns out to be more clear. Embracing a supplement thick eating regimen, participating in standard active work, and keeping up with other way of life factors add to mental save and may diminish the gamble old enough related mental hindrance.

More seasoned grown-ups, confronting the difficulties of maturing and expected mental degradation, can profit from a fair eating regimen wealthy in supplements that help cerebrum wellbeing. Cell reinforcement rich food varieties, omega-3 unsaturated fats, and B-nutrients are especially significant in this phase of life. Furthermore, remaining socially dynamic and intellectually drew in supplements dietary methodologies for keeping up with mental capability.

Natural variables, including financial status and admittance to nutritious food sources, assume a part in forming dietary examples and, therefore, mental and profound prosperity. Variations in admittance to good food sources can add to wholesome lacks and increment the gamble of psychological well-being problems. Tending to these financial determinants is vital for advancing evenhanded open doors for mental and profound wellbeing.

Culinary practices and social inclinations likewise impact dietary decisions. Understanding and regarding social variety in dietary examples is fundamental for advancing wellbeing without forcing one-size-fits-all proposals. Fitting dietary guidance to social settings can upgrade the viability of intercessions pointed toward working on mental capability and close to home security.

All in all, the effect of a fair eating regimen on mental capability and close to home solidness is a diverse and dynamic relationship that traverses across the life expectancy. The supplements we consume assume basic parts in supporting cerebrum wellbeing, impacting synapse balance, safeguarding against oxidative pressure, and regulating the stomach mind hub. Taking on a decent and supplement thick eating routine, alongside other way of life factors, arises as an all encompassing way to deal with advancing ideal mental capability and close to home prosperity. Perceiving the multifaceted exchange among sustenance and psychological wellness gives important experiences to people, medical care experts, and policymakers looking to improve mental capacities and profound flexibility across different populaces.

3.3 Practical tips for maintaining a healthy gut through nutrition.

Keeping a solid stomach is fundamental for in general prosperity, as the stomach assumes a vital part in processing, supplement retention, and safe capability. Research progressively underlines the meaning of a decent and supplement rich eating routine in supporting stomach wellbeing. Down to earth methods for accomplishing and keeping a sound stomach through sustenance envelop various dietary decisions and way of life factors.

Fiber-Rich Food varieties:

Integrating an assortment of fiber-rich food varieties into the eating routine is central for stomach wellbeing. Fiber goes about as a prebiotic, sustaining gainful stomach microorganisms. Entire grains, organic products, vegetables, vegetables, and nuts are astounding wellsprings of fiber. Eating a different scope of plant-based food varieties gives various kinds of fiber that help a flourishing local area of stomach microorganisms.

Probiotic-Rich Food varieties:

Probiotics are valuable live microscopic organisms that present medical advantages to the host. Remembering probiotic-rich food sources for the eating regimen acquaints these gainful microorganisms with the stomach. Matured food varieties like yogurt, kefir, sauerkraut, kimchi, miso, and tempeh are regular wellsprings of probiotics. Customary utilization of these food varieties adds to the variety and equilibrium of the stomach microbiota.

Prebiotic Food sources:

Prebiotics are non-absorbable strands that advance the development and action of useful stomach microbes. Food sources rich in prebiotics incorporate garlic, onions, leeks, asparagus, bananas, and Jerusalem artichokes. Joining prebiotic and probiotic food sources makes a synergistic impact, encouraging a solid stomach climate.

Brilliant Foods grown from the ground:

The lively shades of foods grown from the ground mean the presence of different phytochemicals and cancer prevention agents that advantage stomach wellbeing.

These mixtures assist with lessening aggravation, safeguard against oxidative pressure, and backing the development of valuable stomach microscopic organisms. Hold back nothing exhibit of varieties to guarantee an expansive range of supplements.

Hydration:

Remaining sufficiently hydrated is urgent for keeping up with stomach wellbeing. Water helps in the assimilation and retention of supplements and supports the mucosal coating of the digestion tracts. Lack of hydration can prompt clogging and frustrate legitimate absorption. Hold back nothing day to day water consumption, and consider hydrating food sources like watermelon and cucumber.

Restricting Handled Food sources:

Handled food sources, frequently high in sugar, unfortunate fats, and added substances, can adversely affect the stomach microbiota. These food varieties might add to irritation and disturb the equilibrium of useful microorganisms. Restricting the admission of handled and sweet food varieties is vital to keeping a sound stomach climate.

Entire Food varieties and Supplement Thickness:

Focus on entire food varieties that are supplement thick for ideal stomach wellbeing. Supplement thick food varieties give fundamental nutrients, minerals, and cell reinforcements that help by and large prosperity. Underscore different vegetables, organic products, lean proteins, entire grains, and solid fats to guarantee an expansive range of supplements that benefit the stomach.

Restricting Fake Sugars:

A few fake sugars have been related with changes in stomach microbiota organization. While the proof is as yet advancing, directing the admission of fake sweeteners is fitting. Picking normal sugars with some restraint, like honey or maple syrup, might be an ideal choice.

Careful Eating:

Rehearsing careful eating includes focusing on the eating experience, appreciating flavors, and perceiving yearning and completion signals. Biting food completely upholds processing and supplement assimilation. Moreover, careful eating can assist with overseeing pressure, a variable that impacts the stomach mind hub.

Solid Fats:

Remembering wellsprings of solid fats for the eating routine, like avocados, nuts, seeds, and olive oil, adds to destroy wellbeing. These fats support the uprightness of cell films and are associated with the retention of fat-dissolvable nutrients. Omega-3 unsaturated fats, tracked down in greasy fish, flaxseeds, and pecans, have mitigating properties advantageous for the stomach.

Enhancing Protein Sources:

Fluctuating protein sources guarantees a scope of amino acids and supplements that help in general wellbeing. Integrate lean meats, fish, poultry, vegetables, nuts, and seeds into the eating regimen. Differentiating protein sources likewise adds to a more different stomach microbiota.

Standard, Adjusted Dinners:

Laying out a standard eating design with adjusted dinners upholds stomach capability. Sporadic dietary patterns or outrageous weight control plans can upset the stomach microbiota and influence stomach related processes. Hold back nothing of macronutrients in every feast, including starches, proteins, and sound fats.

Restricting Anti-microbial Use Whenever the situation allows:

Anti-microbials, while vital for treating bacterial diseases, can likewise influence the stomach microbiota. Abuse or pointless utilization of anti-infection agents might prompt aggravations in stomach microorganisms. At the point when endorsed anti-toxins, it's vital to heed clinical guidance and consider probiotic supplementation to help stomach wellbeing.

Active work:

Customary active work has been related with a more different and adjusted stomach microbiota. Practice animates stomach motility, advancing sound assimilation. Integrate both high-impact and obstruction practices into your daily schedule for thorough medical advantages.

Satisfactory Rest:

Quality rest is fundamental for generally wellbeing, including stomach wellbeing. Disturbances in rest examples can impact the stomach microbiota and add to irritation. Go for the gold long stretches of value rest each night to help ideal physical and mental prosperity.

Stress The board:

Constant pressure can adversely affect the stomach cerebrum hub, prompting changes in stomach motility and penetrability. Integrating pressure the board strategies, like contemplation, profound breathing activities, or yoga, can assist with supporting stomach wellbeing.

Food Bigotries:

Distinguishing and tending to food bigotries can be critical for stomach wellbeing. Normal bigotries incorporate lactose and gluten. In the event that you suspect a particular food is causing stomach related issues, consider talking with a medical services proficient or an enlisted dietitian for direction.

Aged Refreshments:

Notwithstanding matured food sources, consolidating matured drinks like fermented tea and kefir can give a wellspring of probiotics. These drinks offer a delectable method for improving stomach wellbeing and enhance the kinds of useful microscopic organisms in the microbiota.

Balance and Assortment:

Control and assortment are key standards for a solid and adjusted diet. Keeping away from inordinate utilization of a specific nutrition class and embracing various food varieties guarantees a wide scope of supplements that help generally speaking wellbeing, including stomach wellbeing.

Talking with a Medical services Proficient:

Individual nourishing necessities can shift in view of elements like age, orientation, wellbeing status, and explicit dietary prerequisites. Talking with a medical services proficient or an enrolled dietitian can give customized direction to improve stomach wellbeing in light of individual necessities and inclinations.

All in all, keeping a solid stomach through nourishment includes a complex methodology that envelops a different and adjusted diet, careful eating practices, and way of life factors. The stomach microbiota, impacted by dietary decisions, assumes a focal part in generally speaking wellbeing, influencing processing, supplement retention, and safe capability. By integrating commonsense tips for stomach wellbeing into day to day existence, people can advance a flourishing stomach microbiota and support their prosperity from the back to front.

Mental capability and close to home strength are basic parts of human prosperity, affecting how people explore their regular routines, associate with others, and adjust to difficulties. The perplexing interaction between mental cycles and profound states shapes one's generally speaking psychological wellness and strength. Understanding the variables that add to mental capability and close to home security is pivotal for advancing ideal mental prosperity and tending to difficulties in emotional well-being.

Mental Capability:

Mental capability alludes to the psychological cycles that empower people to procure, interaction, store, and use data. These cycles envelop a large number of exercises, including insight, consideration, memory, language, critical thinking, and navigation. Mental capability isn't static; it advances all through the life expectancy, impacted by hereditary elements, natural openings, and way of life decisions.

1. **Discernment:**

    Discernment is the capacity to decipher and get a handle on tactile data from the climate. It includes the mind's handling of visual, hear-able, olfactory, gustatory, and material boosts. Discernment is critical for figuring out the world, perceiving objects, and answering fittingly to outside improvements.

2. **Consideration:**

    Consideration is the mental interaction that permits people to zero in on unambiguous boosts while sifting through immaterial data. It assumes a pivotal part in errands requiring fixation, for example, perusing, critical thinking, and learning. Consideration can be specific, maintained, partitioned, or exchanging in view of the requests of the circumstance.

3. **Memory:**

    Memory includes the encoding, stockpiling, and recovery of data. An intricate interaction incorporates transient memory, long haul memory, and working memory. Memory is fundamental for picking up, shaping new affiliations, and reviewing previous encounters. Factors like age, stress, and rest quality can impact memory capability.

4. **Language:**
Language is a center mental capability that empowers correspondence. It includes the capacity to comprehend and create verbally expressed and composed words, as well as to understand and produce complex sentences. Language is urgent for social communications, schooling, and the outflow of contemplations and feelings.

5. **Critical thinking and Direction:**

Critical thinking and direction include the utilization of mental abilities to defeat difficulties and decide. These cycles are fundamental for adjusting to new circumstances, anticipating the future, and exploring complex conditions. Mental adaptability, decisive reasoning, and key arranging add to powerful critical thinking.

Close to home Strength:
Profound security, otherwise called close to home prosperity or profound strength, alludes to a singular's capacity to keep a fair and versatile profound state in spite of confronting stressors or life challenges. Close to home security includes the guideline of feelings, the capacity to quickly return from misfortune, and the ability to encounter a great many feelings without being overpowered.

1. **Feeling Guideline:**
Feeling guideline envelops the cycles people use to impact the span, force, and articulation of their feelings. Powerful feeling guideline permits people to oversee pressure, explore relational connections, and settle on informed choices. Maladaptive feeling guideline procedures can add to profound precariousness.

2. **Stress The board:**
Stress is an unavoidable piece of life, and close to home security includes the capacity to actually adapt to stressors. Sound pressure the board incorporates embracing procedures like care, unwinding strategies, actual work, and looking for social help. Ongoing pressure can affect mental capability and close to home prosperity, making pressure the board significant for generally speaking wellbeing.

3. **Flexibility:**
Flexibility is the ability to return from difficulty and keep up with mental prosperity notwithstanding challenges. Strong people can adjust to evolving conditions, gain from misfortunes, and develop a positive mentality. Flexibility is affected by variables like social help, survival methods, and self-adequacy.

4. **The ability to appreciate people at their core:**

The capacity to appreciate individuals on a deeper level includes the capacity to perceive, comprehend, and deal with one's own feelings, as well as to see and impact the feelings of others. High ability to understand individuals on a deeper level adds to viable correspondence, compassionate connections, and cooperative critical thinking. It assumes a huge part in keeping up with profound security.

Factors Impacting Mental Capability and Close to home Steadiness:

A few elements add to the perplexing interaction between mental capability and profound steadiness. These variables incorporate a blend of hereditary, organic, mental, social, and ecological impacts that shape a person's emotional wellness and prosperity.

1. **Hereditary qualities:**
   Hereditary variables assume a part in forming mental capacities and close to home qualities. The heritability of specific mental capabilities, for example, insight, has been concentrated widely. Likewise, hereditary inclinations can impact a person's close to home disposition, including their helplessness to nervousness, misery, or other state of mind problems.

2. **Neurobiology:**
   The design and capability of the mind are basic to both mental capability and close to home soundness. Synapses, like serotonin, dopamine, and norepinephrine, assume a pivotal part in controlling temperament and mental cycles. Cerebrum districts like the prefrontal cortex, hippocampus, and amygdala are engaged with close to home guideline and mental capabilities.

3. **Natural Openings:**
   Early-valuable encounters, natural openings, and the nature of providing care during youth can affect mental turn of events and close to home prosperity. Unfriendly youth encounters (Pros) have been connected to long haul impacts on psychological wellness, including an expanded gamble of mental weaknesses and personal troubles further down the road.

4. **Way of life Decisions:**
   Way of life decisions, including diet, active work, rest, and substance use, altogether impact mental capability and profound security. A decent eating regimen that supports cerebrum wellbeing, customary activity that upgrades mental capacities, quality rest that advances profound prosperity, and keeping away from substances that impede mental capability all add to ideal psychological well-being.

5. **Social Help:**
   Social associations and strong connections are essential for profound soundness. Positive social collaborations, solid informal organizations, and a feeling of having a place add to profound versatility. Depression and social seclusion, then again, can adversely affect emotional well-being and mental capability.

6. **Schooling and Mental Feeling:**
   Instructive open doors and mental feeling add to the turn of events and support of mental capability. Deep rooted getting the hang of, participating in mentally testing exercises, and chasing after leisure activities that animate the brain advance mental imperativeness and may have defensive impacts against mental degradation.

7. **Emotional wellness Issues:**

Psychological wellness issues, like sadness, tension, bipolar confusion, and schizophrenia, can essentially affect both mental capability and close to home solidness. The connection between psychological wellness and mental capacities is bidirectional, with emotional well-being problems impacting mental capability and mental debilitations adding to inner difficulties.

Reasonable Techniques for Improving Mental Capability and Profound Steadiness:

Working on mental capability and close to home soundness includes taking on commonsense methodologies that address the different variables impacting psychological wellness. These procedures include way of life alterations, mental mediations, close to home guideline strategies, and social commitment.

1. **Solid Eating routine:**
   A supplement thick eating regimen that incorporates various organic products, vegetables, entire grains, lean proteins, and solid fats upholds both mental capability and close to home strength. Omega-3 unsaturated fats, tracked down in greasy fish, flaxseeds, and pecans, have been related with mental advantages and temperament guideline.

2. **Ordinary Actual work:**
   Ordinary activity has been connected to worked on mental capability and close to home prosperity. High-impact practice upgrades blood stream to the mind, advances the development of new neurons, and supports mental cycles. Active work additionally adds to pressure decrease and the arrival of endorphins, further developing temperament.

3. **Quality Rest:**
   Focusing on quality rest is fundamental for mental capability and profound dependability. Rest assumes a urgent part in memory solidification, profound guideline, and generally emotional wellness. Laying out a steady rest schedule, establishing a helpful rest climate, and addressing rest issues add to ideal rest cleanliness.

4. **Stress Decrease Procedures:**
   Integrating pressure decrease procedures into day to day existence can improve profound steadiness. Care contemplation, profound breathing activities,

moderate muscle unwinding, and yoga are compelling techniques for overseeing pressure and advancing close to home flexibility. Customary act of these strategies can emphatically influence mental capability too.

5. **Mental Preparation:**

Participating in mental preparation activities can level up mental skills and backing cerebrum wellbeing. Exercises, for example, puzzles, games, memory activities, and mastering new abilities challenge the cerebrum and advance mental feeling. Deep rooted learning and scholarly interest add to mental imperativeness.

6. **Close to home Guideline Abilities:**

Creating close to home guideline abilities is vital for keeping up with profound security. Mental conduct treatment (CBT) and argumentative conduct treatment (DBT) are remedial methodologies that show people compelling procedures for distinguishing, understanding, and dealing with their feelings. These abilities are significant for exploring life's difficulties.

7. **Social Commitment:**

Developing positive social associations and taking part in significant connections are fundamental for close to home prosperity. Social help gives a support against pressure, lessens sensations of forlornness, and adds to generally life fulfillment. Chipping in, joining clubs, and taking part in local area exercises encourage social commitment.

8. **Long lasting Learning:**

Long lasting learning adds to mental feeling as well as improves by and large prosperity. Seeking after interests, getting new abilities, and remaining mentally connected over the course of life are related with mental versatility. Instructive open doors and interest driven learning add to a satisfying and intellectually dynamic way of life.

9. **Emotional well-being Registrations:**

Ordinary psychological well-being registrations include checking one's close to home prosperity and looking for help when required. Perceiving early indications of stress, uneasiness, or sadness considers convenient mediation. Psychological wellness registrations can be worked with through self-reflection, journaling, or conversations with confided in companions, relatives, or emotional well-being experts.

10. **Proficient Help:**

Looking for proficient help while confronting difficulties in mental capability or profound dependability is a proactive move toward mental prosperity. Emotional wellness experts, including analysts, advocates, and specialists, can give restorative mediations, directing, and, if important, prescription administration.

Chapter 4

Superfoods and Nutrient-Rich Choices

In the steadily advancing scene of sustenance and wellbeing, the expression "superfoods" has acquired significant prominence. These supplement pressed forces to be reckoned with are hailed for their extraordinary medical advantages and high groupings of fundamental nutrients, minerals, and cancer prevention agents. As people become progressively aware of their dietary decisions, the mission for superfoods has turned into a point of convergence chasing ideal prosperity.

One such superfood that has gathered far and wide praise is kale. This verdant green is a dietary force to be reckoned with, plentiful in nutrients A, C, and K, as well as minerals prefer iron and calcium. Kale's flexibility makes it a #1 among wellbeing fans; it tends to be integrated into plates of mixed greens, smoothies, or sautéed dishes. Its powerful flavor and crunchy surface add a magnificent aspect to feasts while adding to a balanced supplement profile.

Berries, as well, have procured their status as superfoods because of their intense cancer prevention agent content. Blueberries, strawberries, raspberries, and blackberries are delectable as well as overflowing with nutrients and phytochemicals that help in general wellbeing. The lively tones of these berries are demonstrative of their high cell reinforcement levels, which assume a urgent part in battling oxidative pressure and lessening irritation in the body.

Quinoa, a without gluten grain, has turned into a staple in numerous wellbeing cognizant families. Loaded with protein, fiber, and a heap of fundamental supplements, quinoa offers a healthy option in contrast to customary grains. Its nutty flavor and somewhat chewy surface make it a flexible fixing in plates of mixed greens, bowls, and side dishes.

Avocados, frequently alluded to as a superfood for their rich monounsaturated fats, are praised for their heart-sound advantages. Past their sound fats, avocados are a decent wellspring of potassium, vitamin K, and folate. The velvety surface and gentle taste of avocados make them a flexible expansion to plates of mixed greens, sandwiches, and smoothies.

Salmon, a greasy fish wealthy in omega-3 unsaturated fats, is another superfood that upholds cardiovascular wellbeing. Omega-3s are fundamental fats that assume a critical part in mind capability and diminishing irritation. Salmon's exquisite taste and flaky surface make it a delightful choice for those looking for a supplement thick protein source.

Chia seeds have arisen as a superfood whiz, known for their noteworthy wholesome profile. Loaded with fiber, protein, and omega-3 unsaturated fats, these minuscule seeds can be handily integrated into different dishes, including yogurt, smoothies, and oats. Chia seeds additionally have the remarkable capacity to retain fluid and make a gel-like consistency, pursuing them a well known decision for making solid puddings and drinks.

Turmeric, a brilliant toned zest, has been utilized for a really long time in customary medication for its mitigating properties. The dynamic compound in turmeric, curcumin, is liable for the vast majority of its medical advantages. Adding turmeric to dishes bestows a warm, natural flavor yet additionally gives a likely lift to the body's capacity to battle irritation.

Salad greens, for example, spinach and Swiss chard are supplement rich decisions that offer a plenty of nutrients and minerals. Loaded with iron, magnesium, and nutrients An and K, these greens add to by and large prosperity and backing different physical processes. Whether sautéed, steamed, or integrated into servings of mixed greens, salad greens are an important expansion to a fair eating routine.

Nuts and seeds, including almonds, pecans, and flaxseeds, are supplement thick choices that give a blend of solid fats, protein, and fundamental nutrients and minerals. These versatile tidbits are advantageous as well as add to satiety and energy levels. Whether delighted in all alone or added to yogurt, mixed greens, or smoothies, nuts and seeds offer a wonderful crunch and a wholesome lift.

Yams, with their energetic orange shade, are a supplement rich option in contrast to standard potatoes. Loaded with beta-carotene, nutrients, and fiber, yams support eye wellbeing, invulnerable capability, and assimilation. Broiled, crushed, or heated, yams are a tasty and nutritious expansion to dinners.

Greek yogurt has acquired fame as a superfood because of its high protein content and probiotic properties. Wealthy in calcium and helpful microorganisms, Greek yogurt upholds stomach related wellbeing and adds to major areas of strength for a framework. Whether delighted in all alone or utilized as a base for smoothies and flavorful dishes, Greek yogurt adds a velvety surface and a healthful lift to different recipes.

Broccoli, a cruciferous vegetable, is a supplement stalwart that gives a wealth of nutrients, minerals, and cell reinforcements. High in L-ascorbic acid, folate, and fiber, broccoli upholds resistant capability and stomach related wellbeing. Its flexible nature considers consideration in sautés, mixed greens, and side dishes.

The medical advantages of green tea have been lauded for quite a long time, and it keeps on being a famous drink decision for those looking for cell reinforcement rich choices. Loaded with catechins, green tea has been connected to different medical advantages, including further developed heart wellbeing and improved digestion. Delighted in hot or cool, green tea gives a reviving and restorative drink choice.

Integrating these superfoods and supplement rich decisions into a reasonable eating routine can add to in general wellbeing and prosperity. Notwithstanding, it's fundamental for approach dietary decisions with an all encompassing point of view, taking into account individual requirements, inclinations, and way of life factors. While superfoods offer a concentrated portion of supplements, a different and balanced diet is critical to guaranteeing that the body gets an expansive range of fundamental nutrients and minerals.

Monotony wears on the soul this turns out as expected in the domain of sustenance. Consuming a different scope of natural products, vegetables, entire grains, lean proteins, and sound fats guarantees that the body gets an expansive cluster of supplements important for ideal working. As opposed to zeroing in exclusively on individual superfoods, embracing an eating routine wealthy in variety can give a thorough nourishing establishment.

It means a lot to take note of that while superfoods can be important increments to a solid eating routine, they ought not be seen as wizardry slugs or convenient solutions. Practical wellbeing is a consequence of steady, long haul way of life decisions that include dietary propensities as well as actual work, sufficient rest, stress the board, and hydration.

Additionally, individual wholesome necessities change in light of variables, for example, age, orientation, action level, and fundamental medical issue. Talking with a medical care proficient or an enrolled dietitian can give customized direction custommade to explicit requirements and objectives. These specialists can offer bits of knowledge into segment sizes, supplement prerequisites, and dietary changes that line up with a singular's remarkable conditions.

All in all, the universe of superfoods and supplement rich decisions is sweeping and different, offering a large number of choices to help a sound way of life. From mixed greens to greasy fish, nuts to berries, each superfood brings its interesting arrangement of supplements and medical advantages to the table. Integrating different these supplement stuffed decisions into an even eating regimen can add to in general prosperity and imperativeness.

Notwithstanding, it's significant to move toward nourishment with an all encompassing outlook, perceiving that a mix of different food sources, alongside other way of life factors, assumes an essential part in keeping up with ideal wellbeing. Superfoods can unquestionably be an important part of a sound eating routine, yet they are best when part of a more extensive methodology that incorporates ordinary active work, adequate rest, and stress the executives.

As people explore the immense range of superfoods and supplement rich decisions accessible, crucial for find some kind of harmony lines up with their preferences, inclinations, and individual healthful requirements. Eventually, a careful and informed way to deal with sustenance, combined with a promise to long haul prosperity, establishes the groundwork for a sound and lively life.

4.1 Identifying and exploring the nutritional benefits of superfoods.

In the consistently developing scene of sustenance and wellbeing, the expression "superfoods" has acquired impressive prevalence. These supplement stuffed forces to be reckoned with are hailed for their excellent medical advantages and high groupings of fundamental nutrients, minerals, and cancer prevention agents. Distinguishing and investigating the healthful advantages of superfoods is an excursion into the different universe of food sources that go past simple food, offering a plenty of supplements that add to by and large prosperity.

One such superfood that has accumulated far and wide recognition is kale. This verdant green is a nourishing force to be reckoned with, plentiful in nutrients A, C, and K, as well as minerals prefer iron and calcium. Kale's flexibility makes it a number one among wellbeing fans; it tends to be integrated into plates of mixed greens, smoothies, or sautéed dishes. Its strong flavor and crunchy surface add a great aspect to feasts while adding to a balanced supplement profile. The high satisfied of cancer prevention agents, including beta-carotene and quercetin, in kale upholds the body's guard against oxidative pressure and irritation.

Berries, as well, have acquired their status as superfoods because of their intense cell reinforcement content. Blueberries, strawberries, raspberries, and blackberries are scrumptious as well as overflowing with nutrients and phytochemicals that help generally speaking wellbeing. The lively tones of these berries are characteristic of their high cell reinforcement levels, which assume a urgent part in fighting oxidative pressure and decreasing irritation in the body. Furthermore, berries contain fiber, which advances stomach related wellbeing and manages glucose levels.

Quinoa, a sans gluten grain, has turned into a staple in numerous wellbeing cognizant families. Loaded with protein, fiber, and a bunch of fundamental supplements, quinoa offers a healthy option in contrast to conventional grains. Its nutty flavor and marginally chewy surface make it a flexible fixing in servings of mixed greens, bowls, and side dishes.

Quinoa is especially prominent for being a finished protein, meaning it gives each of the nine fundamental amino acids that the body can't deliver all alone. This pursues it a fantastic decision for veggie lovers and vegetarians hoping to meet their protein needs.

Avocados, frequently alluded to as a superfood for their rich monounsaturated fats, are commended for their heart-solid advantages. Past their sound fats, avocados are a decent wellspring of potassium, vitamin K, and folate. The rich surface and gentle taste of avocados make them a flexible expansion to servings of mixed greens, sandwiches, and smoothies. The monounsaturated fats in avocados are related with further developed cholesterol levels and cardiovascular wellbeing, making them an important consideration in a heart-sound eating routine.

Salmon, a greasy fish wealthy in omega-3 unsaturated fats, is another superfood that upholds cardiovascular wellbeing. Omega-3s are fundamental fats that assume a pivotal part in mind capability and lessening irritation. Salmon's flavorful taste and flaky surface make it a luscious choice for those looking for a supplement thick protein source. The omega-3 unsaturated fats in salmon, explicitly eicosapentaenoic corrosive (EPA) and docosahexaenoic corrosive (DHA), have been connected to a diminished gamble of coronary illness and worked on mental capability.

Chia seeds have arisen as a superfood genius, known for their great wholesome profile. Loaded with fiber, protein, and omega-3 unsaturated fats, these minuscule seeds can be effectively integrated into different dishes, including yogurt, smoothies, and oats. Chia seeds likewise have the remarkable capacity to retain fluid and make a gel-like consistency, going with them a well known decision for making sound puddings and refreshments. The solvent fiber in chia seeds adds to sensations of completion and helps in absorption, while the omega-3 unsaturated fats support heart wellbeing and mental capability.

Turmeric, a brilliant tinted flavor, has been utilized for a really long time in customary medication for its calming properties. The dynamic compound in turmeric, curcumin, is answerable for the majority of its medical advantages. Adding turmeric to dishes confers a warm, hearty flavor yet in addition gives a likely lift to the body's capacity to battle irritation. Curcumin's mitigating impacts might help conditions like joint pain and may add to in general joint wellbeing. Furthermore, turmeric has cell reinforcement properties that assist with killing free extremists in the body.

Salad greens, for example, spinach and Swiss chard are supplement rich decisions that offer a plenty of nutrients and minerals. Loaded with iron, magnesium, and nutrients An and K, these greens add to generally prosperity and backing different physical processes. Whether sautéed, steamed, or integrated into plates of mixed greens, salad greens are a significant expansion to a fair eating regimen. The iron in spinach, for instance, is fundamental for shipping oxygen all through the body and forestalling iron-lack sickliness.

Nuts and seeds, including almonds, pecans, and flaxseeds, are supplement thick choices that give a blend of sound fats, protein, and fundamental nutrients and minerals. These compact bites are advantageous as well as add to satiety and energy levels. Whether delighted in all alone or added to yogurt, mixed greens, or smoothies, nuts and seeds offer a fantastic crunch and a nourishing lift. Almonds, for example, are plentiful in vitamin E, a cell reinforcement that assumes a part in skin wellbeing and safe capability. Pecans, then again, are a decent wellspring of omega-3 unsaturated fats, which are critical for mind wellbeing.

Yams, with their lively orange tint, are a supplement rich option in contrast to normal potatoes. Loaded with beta-carotene, nutrients, and fiber, yams support eye wellbeing, resistant capability, and absorption. Simmered, pounded, or heated, yams are a flavorful and nutritious expansion to dinners. The beta-carotene in yams is changed over into vitamin An in the body, advancing solid vision and supporting the safe framework.

Greek yogurt has acquired ubiquity as a superfood because of its high protein content and probiotic properties. Wealthy in calcium and useful microscopic organisms, Greek yogurt upholds stomach related wellbeing and adds to major areas of strength for a framework. Whether delighted in all alone or utilized as a base for smoothies and flavorful dishes, Greek yogurt adds a rich surface and a healthful lift to different recipes. The probiotics in Greek yogurt advance a good arrangement of stomach microbes, which is fundamental for stomach related prosperity.

Broccoli, a cruciferous vegetable, is a supplement stalwart that gives an overflow of nutrients, minerals, and cell reinforcements. High in L-ascorbic acid, folate, and fiber, broccoli upholds resistant capability and stomach related wellbeing. Its flexible nature considers consideration in pan-sears, mixed greens, and side dishes. Broccoli contains sulforaphane, a compound with potential enemy of disease properties, and indole-3-carbinol, which might have defensive impacts against specific sorts of malignant growth.

The medical advantages of green tea have been praised for quite a long time, and it keeps on being a well known refreshment decision for those looking for cell reinforcement rich choices. Loaded with catechins, green tea has been connected to different medical advantages, including further developed heart wellbeing and upgraded digestion. Delighted in hot or chilly, green tea gives a reviving and refreshing drink choice. The catechins in green tea, especially epigallocatechin gallate (EGCG), have been read up for their likely job in advancing cardiovascular wellbeing and supporting weight the executives.

Integrating these superfoods and supplement rich decisions into a decent eating regimen can add to generally speaking wellbeing and prosperity. Be that as it may, it's crucial for approach dietary decisions with an all encompassing point of view, taking into account individual necessities, inclinations, and way of life factors.

While superfoods offer a concentrated portion of supplements, a different and balanced diet is critical to guaranteeing that the body gets an expansive range of fundamental nutrients and minerals.

Monotony wears on the soul this turns out as expected in the domain of sustenance. Consuming a different scope of organic products, vegetables, entire grains, lean proteins, and solid fats guarantees that the body gets a wide cluster of supplements vital for ideal working. As opposed to zeroing in exclusively on individual superfoods, embracing an eating regimen wealthy in variety can give a complete dietary establishment.

It means a lot to take note of that while superfoods can be important increments to a solid eating regimen, they ought not be seen as wizardry slugs or convenient solutions. Maintainable wellbeing is a consequence of reliable, long haul way of life decisions that include dietary propensities as well as active work, sufficient rest, stress the board, and hydration.

In addition, individual wholesome requirements shift in view of elements, for example, age, orientation, action level, and fundamental ailments. Talking with a medical care proficient or an enrolled dietitian can give customized direction custommade to explicit requirements and objectives. These specialists can offer experiences into segment sizes, supplement necessities, and dietary changes that line up with a singular's remarkable conditions.

All in all, the universe of superfoods and supplement rich decisions is sweeping and different, offering a huge number of choices to help a solid way of life. From mixed greens to greasy fish, nuts to berries, each superfood brings its remarkable arrangement of supplements and medical advantages to the table. Integrating various these supplement stuffed decisions into an even eating routine can add to in general prosperity and essentialness.

Notwithstanding, it's urgent to move toward nourishment with an all encompassing mentality, perceiving that a mix of different food varieties, alongside other way of life factors, assumes a critical part in keeping up with ideal wellbeing. Superfoods can positively be an important part of a sound eating regimen, yet they are best when part of a more extensive technique that incorporates standard active work, adequate rest, and stress the board.

4.2 Providing a list of nutrient-dense foods that support overall health.

In the domain of sustenance, the journey for ideal wellbeing frequently revolves around devouring supplement thick food sources that give an abundance of fundamental nutrients, minerals, and other useful mixtures. A different and even eating regimen that integrates various supplement thick choices can add to generally speaking prosperity, supporting different physical processes and advancing essentialness. Here, we dive into a complete rundown of supplement thick food sources that act as important increases to a wellbeing cognizant eating routine.

Salad greens, like spinach, kale, and Swiss chard, are healthful forces to be reckoned with that offer a variety of nutrients and minerals. Loaded with iron, calcium, magnesium, and nutrients An and K, these greens add to bone wellbeing, invulnerable capability, and in general imperativeness. The high fiber content guides processing and advances a sensation of totality. These mixed greens are flexible and can be integrated into servings of mixed greens, smoothies, or sautéed dishes, giving a supplement lift to any feast.

Berries, including blueberries, strawberries, raspberries, and blackberries, are delightful as well as plentiful in cancer prevention agents, nutrients, and fiber. The lively shades of berries show their high cell reinforcement content, which helps battle oxidative pressure and aggravation in the body. Berries are likewise a decent wellspring of L-ascorbic acid, supporting invulnerable wellbeing, and their fiber content advances stomach related prosperity. Whether delighted in new, frozen, or added to yogurt and smoothies, berries are a tasty and nutritious decision.

Quinoa, a without gluten entire grain, stands apart for its finished protein profile, containing every one of the nine fundamental amino acids. This makes quinoa a great plant-based protein hotspot for veggie lovers and vegetarians. Furthermore, quinoa is plentiful in fiber, magnesium, iron, and B-nutrients. Its nutty flavor and flexibility go with it a well known decision for plates of mixed greens, bowls, and side dishes, giving a supplement stuffed option in contrast to conventional grains.

Avocados are praised for their monounsaturated fats, which add to heart wellbeing by supporting solid cholesterol levels. Notwithstanding sound fats, avocados give potassium, vitamin K, vitamin E, and folate. The rich surface and gentle flavor make avocados a flexible expansion to servings of mixed greens, sandwiches, and smoothies. The supplement profile of avocados, joined with their satisfying properties, pursues them a fantastic and nutritious decision.

Salmon, a greasy fish, is wealthy in omega-3 unsaturated fats, explicitly EPA (eicosapentaenoic corrosive) and DHA (docosahexaenoic corrosive). These fundamental unsaturated fats assume a pivotal part in mind wellbeing, diminishing irritation, and supporting cardiovascular capability. Salmon is additionally a decent wellspring of great protein, B-nutrients, and minerals like selenium. Barbecued, prepared, or seared, salmon is a luscious and supplement thick protein choice.

Chia seeds have acquired superfood status because of their noteworthy healthful substance. These minuscule seeds are wealthy in fiber, omega-3 unsaturated fats, and plant-based protein. Chia seeds can ingest fluid and make a gel-like consistency, pursuing them a famous decision for puddings, smoothies, and refreshments. The dissolvable fiber in chia seeds advances stomach related wellbeing, while omega-3 unsaturated fats add to heart wellbeing and mental capability.

Turmeric, a brilliant tinted flavor, contains the dynamic compound curcumin, which shows intense calming and cell reinforcement properties. Adding turmeric to dishes bestows a warm, natural flavor yet additionally gives potential medical advantages. Curcumin has been read up for its part in lessening aggravation and may have applications in overseeing conditions like joint pain. Turmeric's cell reinforcement properties assist with killing free revolutionaries in the body.

Nuts and seeds, including almonds, pecans, flaxseeds, and chia seeds, are supplement thick choices that give a blend of sound fats, protein, and fundamental nutrients and minerals. Almonds, for instance, are plentiful in vitamin E, a cancer prevention agent significant for skin wellbeing and safe capability. Pecans are known for their omega-3 unsaturated fat substance, which supports cerebrum wellbeing. Flaxseeds offer a plant-based wellspring of omega-3s and fiber, adding to heart wellbeing and stomach related prosperity. Remembering various nuts and seeds for the eating routine gives a delightful crunch and a large group of healthful advantages.

Yams, with their lively orange tone, are a rich wellspring of beta-carotene, a forerunner to vitamin A. Beta-carotene advances sound vision, skin, and invulnerable capability. Yams additionally give fiber, nutrients C and B6, and minerals like potassium. Simmered, crushed, or prepared, yams offer a heavenly and supplement thick option in contrast to customary potatoes.

Greek yogurt is hailed for its high protein content and probiotic properties. Wealthy in calcium, Greek yogurt upholds bone wellbeing, while its probiotics add to a good arrangement of stomach microscopic organisms. Probiotics are advantageous microorganisms that advance stomach related prosperity and backing the insusceptible framework. Greek yogurt's velvety surface and flexibility make it a brilliant base for both sweet and flavorful dishes, giving a protein-stuffed and probiotic-rich expansion to feasts.

Broccoli, a cruciferous vegetable, is a wholesome force to be reckoned with containing nutrients C and K, folate, fiber, and different cancer prevention agents. Sulforaphane, a compound found in broccoli, has been read up for its potential enemy of disease properties. Furthermore, broccoli upholds insusceptible capability, bone wellbeing, and generally prosperity. Steamed, simmered, or added to plates of mixed greens, broccoli is a flexible and supplement thick vegetable.

Green tea, with its rich history and medical advantages, is a famous drink decision. Loaded with catechins, especially epigallocatechin gallate (EGCG), green tea is known for its cell reinforcement properties. Customary utilization of green tea has been connected to further developed heart wellbeing, upgraded digestion, and possible defensive impacts against specific diseases. Whether delighted in hot or cool, green tea gives a reviving and stimulating drink choice.

Eggs, a total protein source, are plentiful in supplements like choline, vitamin B12, and selenium. The protein in eggs is fundamental for muscle fix and upkeep, while choline upholds cerebrum wellbeing.

Eggs likewise give a scope of fundamental amino acids and are a flexible fixing in different dishes. Bubbled, mixed, or utilized in baking, eggs offer a supplement thick and fulfilling food choice.

Dim chocolate, especially assortments with a high cocoa content, is an astounding expansion to the rundown of supplement thick food sources. Dim chocolate contains cell reinforcements, for example, flavonoids, which have been related with different medical advantages. Also, dull chocolate gives minerals like iron, magnesium, and zinc. Consumed with some restraint, dull chocolate can be a brilliant and stimulating treat.

Spinach, part of the salad greens family, merits extraordinary notice for its remarkable supplement content. Plentiful in iron, calcium, nutrients An and K, and cell reinforcements, spinach upholds generally wellbeing. The iron in spinach is fundamental for oxygen transport in the body, while vitamin K adds to bone wellbeing and blood thickening. Whether added to plates of mixed greens, omelets, or smoothies, spinach is a flexible and supplement thick green.

Oats, an entire grain, are an important wellspring of fiber, especially beta-glucans, which have been connected to heart wellbeing. Oats additionally give complex starches, B-nutrients, and minerals like magnesium. The solvent fiber in oats adds to a sensation of completion and controls glucose levels. Whether delighted in as oats, added to smoothies, or utilized in baking, oats offer a healthy and supplement thick choice.

Cauliflower, a cruciferous vegetable, is low in calories however high in supplements. It contains nutrients C and K, folate, fiber, and different cell reinforcements. Cauliflower is a flexible fixing that can be utilized as a low-carb elective in recipes, for example, cauliflower rice or cauliflower pizza covering. The mixtures in cauliflower, including sulforaphane, add to its potential enemy of disease properties and generally medical advantages.

Tomatoes, wealthy in cell reinforcements like lycopene, are a supplement thick natural product that upholds heart wellbeing. Lycopene has been connected to a decreased gamble of specific diseases and adds to the energetic red shade of tomatoes. Also, tomatoes give nutrients C and K, potassium, and folate. Whether delighted in new in plates of mixed greens, as a base for sauces, or in soups, tomatoes add flavor and sustenance to various dishes.

Ringer peppers, accessible in different tones, are supplement thick vegetables plentiful in nutrients An and C. The dynamic tints of ringer peppers mean their cell reinforcement content, which upholds invulnerable capability and skin wellbeing. Ringer peppers likewise give fiber and are a flexible fixing in plates of mixed greens, pan-sears, and fajitas. Counting different varieties adds visual allure and a different scope of supplements.

Salad greens, past the usually referenced spinach and kale, incorporate various supplement thick choices like arugula, romaine lettuce, and watercress.

These greens offer a blend of nutrients, minerals, and cell reinforcements that add to by and large wellbeing. Integrating an assortment of salad greens into dinners gives a different scope of supplements and flavors.

Cabbage, another cruciferous vegetable, is low in calories however high in supplements. Plentiful in nutrients C and K, as well as fiber and cancer prevention agents, cabbage upholds stomach related wellbeing and safe capability. Whether utilized in coleslaw, sautés, or soups, cabbage is a flexible and supplement thick expansion to a wellbeing cognizant eating routine.

Mushrooms, like shiitake, maitake, and clam mushrooms, are tasty as well as supplement thick. Mushrooms give nutrients like D and B-nutrients, as well as minerals can imagine selenium. The high fiber content in mushrooms upholds stomach related wellbeing. Whether sautéed, barbecued, or added to soups, mushrooms contribute an extraordinary umami flavor and wholesome .

4.3 Recipes and meal ideas incorporating these superfoods into daily meals.

Coordinating superfoods into day to day dinners can be a great and compensating culinary experience. These supplement stuffed fixings add to in general wellbeing as well as add flavor, surface, and assortment to a reasonable eating routine. We should investigate a few imaginative recipes and dinner thoughts that consolidate superfoods, transforming standard feasts into remarkable nourishing forces to be reckoned with.

1. **Quinoa and Veggie Buddha Bowl:**
   Begin with a base of cooked quinoa, a total protein source. Top it with a bright cluster of cooked yams, cherry tomatoes, sautéed kale, and cut avocado. Shower with a tahini dressing for added smoothness and flavor. This Buddha Bowl gives an equilibrium of macronutrients, nutrients, and minerals in an outwardly engaging and fulfilling dish.

2. **Salmon and Berry Salad:**
   Consolidate the extravagance of omega-3 unsaturated fats from barbecued or heated salmon with the cell reinforcement force of blended berries. Make a lively plate of mixed greens by throwing spinach or blended greens in with cut strawberries, blueberries, and raspberries. Top with barbecued salmon filets and a light vinaigrette made with olive oil, balsamic vinegar, and a bit of honey.

3. **Chia Seed Pudding Parfait:**
   Make a nutritious and delectable chia seed pudding by drenching chia seeds in almond milk for the time being. Layer the pudding with Greek yogurt and a variety of new berries in a glass or bowl. Top with a sprinkle of granola and a shower of honey for added crunch and pleasantness. This parfait is a fantastic breakfast or sound pastry choice.

4. **Turmeric-mixed Lentil Soup:**
   Improve the calming properties of turmeric by integrating it into a good lentil soup. Sauté onions, garlic, carrots, and celery in olive oil, then, at that point, add lentils, vegetable stock, and turmeric. Stew until the lentils are delicate, and wrap up with a press of lemon juice for brilliance. This supporting soup is a consoling and nutritious dinner.

5. **Avocado and Chickpea Wrap:**
   Pound ready avocados and spread them on an entire grain wrap. Add a layer of chickpea salad made with canned chickpeas, cherry tomatoes, cucumber, red onion, and cilantro. Sprinkle with olive oil and a crush of lemon juice prior to wrapping it up. This fast and simple recipe makes for a fantastic lunch with a decent equilibrium of solid fats, fiber, and protein.

6. **Berry and Almond Smoothie Bowl:**
   Mix a smoothie utilizing blended berries, a banana, Greek yogurt, and almond

milk until rich. Empty the smoothie into a bowl and top it with cut almonds, chia seeds, and extra berries. This smoothie bowl isn't just outwardly engaging yet additionally gives an eruption of cell reinforcements, nutrients, and minerals.

7. **Kale and Quinoa Stuffed Peppers:**
Consolidate cooked quinoa with sautéed kale, diced tomatoes, dark beans, and flavors. Slice chime peppers down the middle and eliminate the seeds, then, at that point, stuff them with the quinoa combination. Prepare until the peppers are delicate. Embellish with new cilantro and a touch of Greek yogurt for a nutritious and delightful dinner.

8. **Yam and Chickpea Curry:**
Make a generous and tasty curry by stewing yams, chickpeas, spinach, and diced tomatoes in coconut milk. Add curry flavors like turmeric, cumin, and coriander for a sweet-smelling mix of flavors. Serve over earthy colored rice or quinoa for a total and fulfilling feast.

9. **Pecan and Spinach Pesto Pasta:**
Set up an energetic pesto by mixing spinach, basil, pecans, garlic, Parmesan cheddar, and olive oil. Throw the pesto with entire grain pasta and add cherry tomatoes, sautéed mushrooms, and barbecued chicken for protein. This dish offers a supplement rich bend on an exemplary pasta recipe.

10. **Greek Yogurt Parfait with Granola and Berries:**
Layer Greek yogurt with granola and a blend of new berries for a fast and nutritious parfait. The yogurt gives protein and probiotics, while the granola adds crunch and entire grains. This parfait is a flexible choice for breakfast, a bite, or a solid treat.

11. **Broccoli and Salmon Pan fried food:**
Sauté broccoli florets, chime peppers, and snap peas in a wok with sesame oil and minced garlic. Add reduced down bits of salmon and pan fried food until prepared through. Season with soy sauce, ginger, and a sprinkle of sesame seeds. Serve over earthy colored rice or quinoa for a supplement pressed pan sear.

12. **Kale and Berry Smoothie:**
Mix kale leaves with blended berries, banana, almond milk, and a scoop of protein powder for a nutritious and stimulating smoothie. This green smoothie is a helpful method for pressing in nutrients, cell reinforcements, and fiber, making it a fantastic breakfast or post-exercise choice.

13. **Heated Yam Fries with Avocado Plunge:**
Cut yams into fries, throw them in olive oil, and heat until firm. Set up a straightforward avocado plunge utilizing squashed avocados, lime juice, garlic, and a touch of salt. These heated yam fries with avocado plunge make for a healthy and fulfilling bite or side dish.

14. **Spinach and Feta Stuffed Chicken Bosom:**
Butterfly chicken bosoms and stuff them with a combination of sautéed

spinach, feta cheddar, and sun-dried tomatoes. Prepare until the chicken is cooked through. This dish gives lean protein as well as integrates the flavors and supplements of spinach and tomatoes.

15. **Green Tea-injected Quinoa Salad:**

Mix green tea and use it to cook quinoa, injecting the grains with cancer prevention agents. Throw the cooked quinoa with diced cucumber, cherry tomatoes, feta cheddar, and a shower of olive oil. This invigorating quinoa salad is a nutritious and hydrating choice for a light lunch or side dish.

16. **Almond and Berry For the time being Oats:**

Join moved oats with almond milk, chia seeds, and a blend of berries in a container. Allow it to sit in the fridge short-term, permitting the oats to retain the fluid and mellow. Toward the beginning of the day, top the short-term oats with cut almonds for added crunch. This make-ahead breakfast is a helpful and nutritious choice.

17. **Barbecued Veggie and Hummus Wrap:**

Barbecue a variety of vegetables, for example, zucchini, ringer peppers, and eggplant. Spread an entire grain wrap with hummus and layer the barbecued veggies inside. Roll it up for a fantastic and fiber-rich wrap that joins the kinds of barbecued vegetables and velvety hummus.

18. **Blueberry and Pecan Salad:**

Prepare a serving of mixed greens with blended greens, new blueberries, disintegrated feta cheddar, and toasted pecans.
Sprinkle with a balsamic vinaigrette for a wonderful blend of sweet, flavorful, and crunchy components. This salad makes for an invigorating and supplement thick side dish.

19. **Mango and Avocado Salsa:**

Join diced mango, avocado, red onion, cilantro, and lime juice to make a lively salsa. Use it as a garnish for barbecued chicken or fish, or appreciate it with entire grain tortilla chips as a delightful and supplement stuffed nibble.

20. **Spinach and Feta Omelet:**

Whisk together eggs and empty them into a hot skillet. Add a small bunch of new spinach and disintegrated feta cheddar aside of the omelet prior to collapsing it over. This fast and protein-rich breakfast choice integrates the nutrients and minerals of spinach and the flavorful decency of feta.

Coordinating superfoods into day to day feasts is an extraordinary way to deal with upgrading nourishing admission and advancing generally wellbeing. Superfoods, perceived for their remarkable supplement thickness and medical advantages, offer a different scope of choices to hoist the nourishing profile of your feasts. From supplement stuffed salad greens to cell reinforcement rich berries, protein-pressed seeds, and omega-3-rich fish, consolidating these superfoods into day to day feasts can be a flavorful and remunerating try.

Salad Greens:

Salad greens, like spinach, kale, and Swiss chard, are dietary forces to be reckoned with that can be flawlessly incorporated into different feasts. Think about beginning your day with a supplement loaded green smoothie by mixing kale with banana, berries, and Greek yogurt. For lunch, make an energetic serving of mixed greens with a blend of spinach, arugula, and romaine lettuce, finished off with barbecued chicken or chickpeas, cherry tomatoes, avocado, and a sprinkle of olive oil. At supper, sautéed Swiss chard can be a tasty side dish, supplementing proteins like salmon or tofu.

Berries:

Berries, including blueberries, strawberries, raspberries, and blackberries, add an eruption of variety, flavor, and nourishment to dinners. For breakfast, mix new berries into oats, yogurt, or oat. As an early in the day or evening nibble, partake in a bowl of blended berries in with a small bunch of nuts for a wonderful and stimulating treat. Berries can likewise be integrated into plates of mixed greens, treats, or as a fixing for entire grain flapjacks or waffles, giving cell reinforcements, nutrients, and normal pleasantness.

Quinoa:

Quinoa, a flexible and complete protein source, can be an establishment for various feasts. Set up a quinoa salad by blending cooked quinoa with diced vegetables, feta cheddar, olives, and a lemon vinaigrette.

Quinoa can likewise act as a supplement rich base for grain bowls, pan-sears, or stuffed chime peppers. Its nutty flavor and marginally crunchy surface make it a fantastic option in contrast to customary grains, offering a significant portion of protein, fiber, and fundamental amino acids.

Salmon:

Salmon, wealthy in omega-3 unsaturated fats, is a superfood that upholds heart wellbeing and gives great protein. Barbecue or prepare salmon filets and serve them with a side of cooked yams and steamed broccoli for a balanced and nutritious supper. Integrate chipped salmon into plates of mixed greens, wraps, or grain bowls for an increase in omega-3s. Counting greasy fish like salmon in your week by week feasts adds to cerebrum capability, lessens aggravation, and supports in general cardiovascular prosperity.

Chia Seeds:

Chia seeds are little forces to be reckoned with loaded with fiber, omega-3 unsaturated fats, and fundamental supplements. Make a chia seed pudding by joining chia seeds with almond milk, a hint of honey, and vanilla concentrate. Allow it to sit for the time being to accomplish a pudding-like consistency. Top the pudding with new berries and a sprinkle of nuts for a supplement thick and fulfilling pastry or breakfast choice. Chia seeds can likewise be added to smoothies, yogurt, or oats for an extra wholesome lift.

Avocado:

Avocado, known for its rich surface and solid monounsaturated fats, can raise both flavorful and sweet dishes. Crush avocado on entire grain toast and top it with poached eggs for a supplement pressed breakfast. Make a reviving avocado and mango salsa to go with barbecued chicken or fish. Integrate avocado cuts into servings of mixed greens, wraps, or sandwiches for a portion of heart-solid fats, nutrients, and minerals.

Turmeric:

Turmeric, with its dynamic compound curcumin, flaunts mitigating and cell reinforcement properties. Integrate turmeric into appetizing dishes like curries, stews, or simmered vegetables. Make a brilliant turmeric latte by mixing turmeric with almond milk, ginger, and a smidgen of honey for a relieving and empowering drink. Adding turmeric to dinners improves flavor as well as adds to lessening aggravation in the body.

Mixed Greens:

Mixed greens, like spinach, kale, and Swiss chard, are healthful forces to be reckoned with that can be consistently incorporated into different feasts. Think about beginning your day with a supplement loaded green smoothie by mixing kale with banana, berries, and Greek yogurt. For lunch, make a dynamic serving of mixed greens with a blend of spinach, arugula, and romaine lettuce, finished off with barbecued chicken or chickpeas, cherry tomatoes, avocado, and a shower of olive oil. At supper, sautéed Swiss chard can be a delightful side dish, supplementing proteins like salmon or tofu.

Berries:

Berries, including blueberries, strawberries, raspberries, and blackberries, add an explosion of variety, flavor, and nourishment to dinners. For breakfast, mix new berries into oats, yogurt, or cereal. As an early in the day or evening nibble, partake in a bowl of blended berries in with a modest bunch of nuts for a delightful and empowering treat. Berries can likewise be integrated into plates of mixed greens, treats, or as a garnish for entire grain flapjacks or waffles, giving cell reinforcements, nutrients, and normal pleasantness.

Quinoa:

Quinoa, a flexible and complete protein source, can be an establishment for various feasts. Set up a quinoa salad by blending cooked quinoa with diced vegetables, feta cheddar, olives, and a lemon vinaigrette. Quinoa can likewise act as a supplement rich base for grain bowls, sautés, or stuffed ringer peppers. Its nutty flavor and somewhat crunchy surface make it a superb option in contrast to customary grains, offering a significant portion of protein, fiber, and fundamental amino acids.

Salmon:

Salmon, wealthy in omega-3 unsaturated fats, is a superfood that upholds heart wellbeing and gives excellent protein. Barbecue or heat salmon filets and serve them with a side of broiled yams and steamed broccoli for a balanced and nutritious supper. Integrate chipped salmon into servings of mixed greens, wraps, or grain bowls for an increase in omega-3s. Counting greasy fish like salmon in your week by week feasts adds to mind capability, diminishes aggravation, and supports generally speaking cardiovascular prosperity.

Chia Seeds:

Chia seeds are minuscule forces to be reckoned with loaded with fiber, omega-3 unsaturated fats, and fundamental supplements. Make a chia seed pudding by joining chia seeds with almond milk, a bit of honey, and vanilla concentrate. Allow it to sit for the time being to accomplish a pudding-like consistency. Top the pudding with new berries and a sprinkle of nuts for a supplement thick and fulfilling sweet or breakfast choice. Chia seeds can likewise be added to smoothies, yogurt, or cereal for an extra healthful lift.

Avocado:

Avocado, known for its rich surface and sound monounsaturated fats, can raise both exquisite and sweet dishes. Crush avocado on entire grain toast and top it with poached eggs for a supplement stuffed breakfast. Make a reviving avocado and mango salsa to go with barbecued chicken or fish. Integrate avocado cuts into servings of mixed greens, wraps, or sandwiches for a portion of heart-sound fats, nutrients, and minerals.

Turmeric:

Turmeric, with its dynamic compound curcumin, flaunts calming and cancer prevention agent properties. Integrate turmeric into flavorful dishes like curries, stews, or cooked vegetables.

Make a brilliant turmeric latte by mixing turmeric with almond milk, ginger, and a touch of honey for a relieving and empowering drink. Adding turmeric to dinners upgrades flavor as well as adds to lessening irritation in the body.

Nuts and Seeds:

Nuts and seeds, including almonds, pecans, flaxseeds, and chia seeds, offer a blend of solid fats, protein, and fundamental supplements. Make a supplement thick tidbit by joining blended nuts in with dried berries. Sprinkle chia seeds on top of yogurt or integrate them into natively constructed granola. Add cleaved pecans to plates of mixed greens, oats, or Greek yogurt for a wonderful crunch and an increase in omega-3 unsaturated fats.

Yams:

Yams, with their dynamic orange tone, are plentiful in beta-carotene, nutrients, and fiber. Cook yam wedges and serve them as a side dish or integrate them into Buddha bowls. Squash yams and top them with dark beans, avocado, and salsa for a nutritious and beautiful bend on exemplary pureed potatoes. Yams furnish a characteristic pleasantness alongside a scope of nutrients and minerals.

Greek Yogurt:

Greek yogurt is a protein-rich and probiotic-pressed dairy item that can be delighted in different ways. Begin your day with a parfait by layering Greek yogurt with granola, new berries, and a sprinkle of honey. Utilize Greek yogurt as a base for smoothies to add richness and a protein support. Integrate it into flavorful dishes as a better choice to sharp cream, upgrading the healthful substance of plunges and dressings.

Broccoli:

Broccoli, a cruciferous vegetable, is a supplement thick choice that can be effectively integrated into feasts. Steam or meal broccoli florets and add them to servings of mixed greens, pasta dishes, or sautés. Make a broccoli and cheddar stuffed heated potato for a consoling and nutritious dinner. Broccoli gives an abundance of nutrients, minerals, and cell reinforcements, adding to safe wellbeing and generally prosperity.

Green Tea:

Green tea, eminent for its cell reinforcement content, is a superfood refreshment that can be delighted in over the course of the day. Mix green tea and serve it as a reviving chilled refreshment or a warm cup toward the beginning of the day. Utilize green tea as a base for smoothies, imbuing them with its stimulating properties. Green tea can likewise be integrated into cooking, for example, involving it as a fluid for quinoa or rice, conferring an unpretentious flavor and potential medical advantages.

Eggs:

Eggs are a flexible and supplement thick protein source that can be delighted in different arrangements. Set up a vegetable omelet for breakfast by adding spinach, tomatoes, and ringer peppers. Bubble eggs and cut them onto servings of mixed greens or entire grain toast. Poach eggs and serve them over sautéed greens for a basic and nutritious dinner. Eggs give fundamental supplements, including choline, vitamin B12, and great protein.

Dim Chocolate:

Dim chocolate, with a high cocoa content, can be relished as a liberal yet energizing treat. Pick dim chocolate with somewhere around 70% cocoa for greatest advantages. Partake in a piece of dim chocolate all alone or integrate it into recipes, for example, energy balls, yogurt parfaits, or trail blend. Dull chocolate contains flavonoids with cell reinforcement properties, offering potential cardiovascular advantages when consumed with some restraint.

Spinach:

Spinach, a verdant green, is a flexible superfood that can be coordinated into various dishes. Add new spinach to smoothies for an additional supplement help. Sauté spinach with garlic and olive oil as a basic and nutritious side dish. Integrate spinach into omelets, frittatas, or lasagna for a delightful and supplement pressed expansion.

Spinach gives iron, nutrients An and K, and cell reinforcements, supporting different parts of wellbeing.

Oats:

Oats, an entire grain, are a healthy and fiber-rich choice that can be delighted in various ways. Get ready oats with almond milk, finished off with cut bananas, nuts, and a shower of honey. Make for the time being oats by absorbing oats yogurt and refrigerating them with berries and chia seeds. Integrate oats into baking recipes for better renditions of treats, biscuits, or energy bars. Oats offer supported energy and add to heart wellbeing.

Cauliflower:

Cauliflower, a cruciferous vegetable, is a flexible superfood that can be changed into different culinary manifestations. Make cauliflower rice by beating cauliflower in a food processor and sautéing it as a low-carb elective. Make cauliflower pizza hull for a nutritious and sans gluten pizza base. Meal or pound cauliflower and integrate it into goulashes, soups, or as a side dish. Cauliflower gives nutrients, fiber, and cancer prevention agents, supporting stomach related wellbeing and in general health.

Tomatoes:

Tomatoes, wealthy in lycopene and different cell reinforcements, are a tasty superfood that upgrades the flavor of many dishes. Set up an exemplary Caprese salad with cut tomatoes, new mozzarella, and basil. Make a custom made pureed tomatoes for pasta dishes, pizzas, or as a base for soups.

Appreciate cherry tomatoes as a bite or add them to servings of mixed greens for an explosion of pleasantness. Tomatoes add to heart wellbeing, skin wellbeing, and may offer assurance against specific tumors.

Ringer Peppers:

Ringer peppers, accessible in different varieties, are supplement thick vegetables that add crunch and energy to dinners. Cut chime peppers and plunge them into hummus or Greek yogurt for a fantastic tidbit. Remember diced chime peppers for omelets, pan-sears, or quinoa servings of mixed greens for added flavor and sustenance. Ringer peppers are plentiful in nutrients An and C, cancer prevention agents that help safe capability and skin wellbeing.

Salad Greens:

Salad greens, past the regularly referenced spinach and kale, offer a scope of choices like arugula, romaine lettuce, and watercress. Blend different serving of mixed greens to make a supplement pressed base for servings of mixed greens. Mix it up of brilliant vegetables, nuts, seeds, and a lean protein source to make a balanced feast. Explore different avenues regarding custom made dressings utilizing olive oil.

Chapter 5

Navigating Dietary Trends

In the consistently developing scene of nourishment, dietary patterns travel every which way, each encouraging a way to further developed wellbeing and prosperity. From antiquated ways of thinking to current crazes, people look for direction on what to eat and how to structure their weight control plans. As the world turns out to be progressively interconnected, the progression of data and social impacts shape the manner in which individuals see food and sustenance. Exploring through these dietary patterns requires a nuanced comprehension of the logical proof, social settings, and individual necessities.

By and large, dietary examples have been well established in social practices and nearby accessibility of food. Customary weight control plans frequently mirror the rural practices, environment, and topographical highlights of a district. Notwithstanding, effortlessly of transportation, food decisions have become more different and interconnected. This has brought about the osmosis of different dietary ways of thinking and the rise of worldwide dietary patterns.

One of the unmistakable dietary patterns that has acquired broad consideration is the idea of plant-based eating. Advocates contend that plant-based counts calories are useful for individual wellbeing as well as for the climate. The accentuation is on consuming organic products, vegetables, grains, vegetables, and nuts while limiting or wiping out creature items. Advocates of plant-based abstains from food frequently refer to studies connecting them to diminished hazard of ongoing infections, including coronary illness and specific kinds of malignant growth.

On the other side, pundits call attention to potential wholesome lacks related with elite plant-based eats less carbs, for example, deficient admission of fundamental supplements like vitamin B12, iron, and omega-3 unsaturated fats. The discussion over plant-based eats less features the intricacy of nourishment and the requirement for cautious thought of individual wellbeing necessities.

As of late, irregular fasting has arisen as another famous dietary pattern. This approach includes cycling between times of eating and fasting, with different conventions considering different time windows of food utilization. Defenders of irregular fasting guarantee advantages like weight reduction, worked on metabolic wellbeing, and expanded life span. A few examinations recommend that irregular fasting might impact cell fix cycles and upgrade the body's capacity to adjust to pressure.

In spite of these possible advantages, irregular fasting isn't reasonable for everybody. People with specific ailments, like diabetes or dietary problems, may have to move toward fasting with alert. Moreover, the drawn out impacts of irregular fasting on wellbeing are as yet being examined, and its maintainability as a direction for living remaining parts a subject of progressing research.

The ketogenic diet is one more dietary pattern that possibly affects weight reduction. This high-fat, low-sugar diet plans to prompt a condition of ketosis, where the body depends on ketones for energy rather than glucose. Advocates contend that the ketogenic diet can prompt fast weight reduction and worked on metabolic markers. In any case, concerns have been raised about its drawn out impacts on cardiovascular wellbeing and the potential for supplement lacks because of the confined food decisions.

As people explore these dietary patterns, it is fundamental to think about the possible advantages as well as the dangers and individual varieties. One size doesn't fit all with regards to sustenance, and what works for one individual may not be appropriate for another. Factors, for example, age, orientation, action level, and hidden medical issue assume a significant part in deciding dietary necessities.

The job of hereditary qualities in molding individual reactions to various weight control plans is an area of developing interest in nourishment research. Customized nourishment, in light of hereditary data, means to fit dietary suggestions to a singular's exceptional hereditary cosmetics. While this field is still in its beginning phases, it holds the commitment of giving more exact and successful dietary direction later on.

Amidst dietary patterns and wholesome discussions, the significance of a decent and fluctuated diet ought not be disregarded. The Mediterranean eating regimen, for instance, has reliably been commended for its accentuation on entire food varieties, including natural products, vegetables, olive oil, and lean proteins. This conventional eating regimen is related with various medical advantages, including decreased hazard of cardiovascular illness and further developed life span.

The Mediterranean eating routine fills in as an update that an all encompassing way to deal with sustenance, taking into account the general dietary example as opposed to disconnected parts, is pivotal for wellbeing. It accentuates the meaning of way of life factors, for example, normal actual work and social associations, in advancing prosperity. This coordinated point of view difficulties the reductionist methodology frequently found chasing after disengaged supplements or wizardry food varieties.

In the time of data over-burden, isolating proof based sustenance counsel from sensationalized cases can challenge. Virtual entertainment, with its fast dispersal of patterns and tales, has turned into a critical powerhouse in forming dietary decisions.

VIPs and forces to be reckoned with frequently underwrite explicit weight control plans, adding to their notoriety and making a need to keep moving to attempt the most recent dietary frenzy.

Notwithstanding, established researchers underlines the significance of decisive reasoning and an insightful way to deal with nourishment data. Studies might be misjudged or taken outside any connection to the issue at hand, and the subtleties of exploration discoveries can be lost in the interpretation from logical diaries to traditional press. It is fundamental to depend on trustworthy sources and counsel qualified medical care experts or enrolled dietitians for customized guidance.

The idea of "clean eating" is one more pattern that has gotten some forward momentum lately. This approach empowers the utilization of entire, natural food varieties while staying away from or limiting handled and refined choices. Clean eating is frequently connected with an emphasis on food quality, manageability, and careful eating rehearses. While the expectation behind clean eating is honorable, it can at times prompt prohibitive ways of behaving and an excessively inflexible way to deal with food decisions.

Orthorexia nervosa, a term begat to depict a fixation on good dieting, features the expected traps of taking clean eating to a limit. People with orthorexia may become focused on the immaculateness of their food decisions, prompting nervousness and social separation. Finding some kind of harmony between focusing on nutritious food varieties and keeping an adaptable and pleasant way to deal with eating is critical for generally speaking prosperity.

In the journey for dietary flawlessness, it is fundamental to perceive that food isn't simply fuel; it is likewise a wellspring of delight, culture, and social association. The delight of imparting a dinner to friends and family, the experience of enjoying flavors, and the social meaning of specific food varieties ought not be forfeited in that frame of mind of a glorified eating regimen. Accomplishing a sound connection with food includes finding an equilibrium that feeds both the body and the spirit.

The impact of the food business on dietary patterns can't be disregarded. Showcasing methodologies, item naming, and the accessibility of handled food varieties add to the forming of buyer decisions. Terms like "superfood" and "utilitarian food varieties" are in many cases used to advertise explicit items as having unprecedented medical advantages. While certain food varieties are to be sure supplement thick and proposition wellbeing advancing properties, moving toward such cases with a basic eye is vital.

The effect of financial elements on dietary examples is a significant thought in the conversation of nourishment. Admittance to new, nutritious food sources might be restricted in specific networks, prompting differences in wellbeing results.

The expense of natural or specialty items, frequently connected with wellbeing centered eats less, may put an extra weight on people with lower livelihoods. Tending to these imbalances requires a multi-layered approach, including strategy changes, local area drives, and instruction on reasonable and nutritious food decisions.

The idea of careful eating has acquired notoriety as an offset to the quick moving, occupied dietary patterns pervasive in current culture. Careful eating includes focusing on the tactile parts of eating, like taste, surface, and smell, while monitoring appetite and completion signals. This approach supports a more deliberate and charming relationship with food, encouraging a more noteworthy appreciation for the eating experience.

Social variety assumes a critical part in molding dietary inclinations and practices. Conventional weight control plans, went down through ages, frequently reflect social qualities, strict convictions, and culinary customs. Investigating and commending the variety of worldwide foods can widen one's sense of taste and add to a more comprehensive comprehension of nourishment.

Lately, the discussion over the ecological effect of food decisions has acquired conspicuousness. The carbon impression of various dietary examples, especially the creation of creature items, has ignited conversations about manageable eating. A few people decide to decrease their meat utilization or pick plant-based options as a method for diminishing their ecological effect. While economical eating is a praiseworthy objective, it is fundamental to think about the more extensive picture, including the ecological effect of plant horticulture and transportation.

The intricacy of dietary patterns is additionally intensified by the convergence of nourishment with psychological well-being. Arising research recommends a bidirectional connection among diet and mental prosperity. The stomach mind hub, interfacing the stomach related framework with the focal sensory system, assumes a part in this perplexing association. Certain dietary examples, like the Mediterranean eating routine, have been related with a lower chance of gloom and mental degradation.

Alternately, psychological well-being conditions can impact dietary decisions, frequently prompting close to home or stress-related eating. Understanding the transaction among sustenance and emotional wellness is an advancing field with suggestions for both preventive and remedial mediations. Integrating psychological well-being contemplations into conversations about dietary patterns is essential for advancing all encompassing prosperity.

As people explore the labyrinth of dietary patterns, cultivating a feeling of independence and self-compassion is significant. The strain to adjust to a specific eating routine or accomplish a particular self-perception can add to cluttered eating designs and adversely influence psychological wellness.

A more comprehensive and empathetic way to deal with wellbeing and nourishment perceives that prosperity is diverse and can't be diminished to a bunch of unbending standards.

All in all, exploring dietary patterns requires a smart and informed approach that thinks about individual necessities, social impacts, and the developing scene of sustenance science. The mission for ideal wellbeing ought to be directed by a harmony between proof based suggestions and an appreciation for the different and individual nature of dietary decisions. Embracing a comprehensive perspective on nourishment, including physical and mental prosperity, can prompt a more economical and satisfying way to deal with food and way of life. As the excursion through the universe of dietary patterns proceeds, the vital lies in remaining liberal, fundamentally assessing data, and finding a way that lines up with individual qualities and goals for a solid, dynamic life.

5.1 Analyzing popular dietary trends and their potential benefits and drawbacks.

The domain of nourishment is a unique scene, set apart by a persistent recurring pattern of dietary patterns. From old practices attached in social customs to present day, experimentally supported approaches, people look for direction on the most ideal ways of feeding their bodies. The journey for a better way of life has led to a huge number of dietary patterns, each encouraging novel advantages. In any case, close by the possible benefits, it is critical to examine the downsides and think about the singular subtleties that shape the adequacy of these patterns.

One unavoidable pattern that has caught the public's consideration as of late is the shift towards plant-based eating. Backers of plant-based counts calories contend that they offer a heap of medical advantages, going from weight the board to a diminished gamble of constant illnesses. At its center, a plant-based diet stresses the utilization of entire, plant-determined food sources like organic products, vegetables, grains, vegetables, and nuts, while limiting or barring creature items.

The expected advantages of plant-based slims down are upheld by a developing group of exploration. Studies propose that such weight control plans are related with lower paces of coronary illness, hypertension, and specific kinds of disease. Moreover, plant-based eating is frequently connected to positive ecological results, as it normally requires less assets and produces lower ozone depleting substance discharges contrasted with customary omnivorous eating regimens.

In any case, the progress to a plant-based diet isn't without challenges. Pundits feature potential wholesome lacks related with the avoidance of creature items, like vitamin B12, iron, and omega-3 unsaturated fats.

Vitamin B12, specifically, is essentially tracked down in creature items, and its lack can prompt neurological and hematological problems. Hence, people embracing a plant-based diet should be careful about getting these supplements through braced food sources or enhancements.

Irregular fasting has arisen as another unmistakable dietary pattern, catching the interest of those looking for weight reduction and worked on metabolic wellbeing. This approach includes cycling between times of eating and fasting, with different conventions directing the length of fasting and eating windows. Advocates of discontinuous fasting contend that it can prompt fat misfortune, further developed insulin responsiveness, and other metabolic advantages.

Research on discontinuous fasting is as yet developing, however a few investigations propose that it might set off cell fix cycles and upgrade the body's capacity to adjust to pressure. Notwithstanding, the drawn out impacts of irregular fasting stay unsure, and its reasonableness for all people is a subject of progressing research. Certain populaces, like those with diabetes or a background marked by dietary problems, may have to move toward discontinuous fasting circumspectly, as it could have potentially negative results on their wellbeing.

The ketogenic diet, portrayed by its high-fat and low-starch structure, has acquired prominence for its implied viability in weight reduction and metabolic enhancements. The ketogenic diet means to initiate a condition of ketosis, where the body depends on ketones for energy rather than glucose. Advocates guarantee that this change in digestion can prompt quick weight reduction and further developed insulin awareness.

While certain investigations support the transient adequacy of the ketogenic diet for weight reduction, concerns have been raised about its possible long haul influence on cardiovascular wellbeing. The eating regimen's high immersed fat substance might raise cholesterol levels, presenting expected dangers to heart wellbeing. Moreover, the prohibitive idea of the eating regimen might bring about supplement lacks and difficulties in keeping up with dietary adherence over the long haul.

As people explore through these dietary patterns, the significance of customized nourishment turns out to be progressively obvious. The possibility that one size fits all in the domain of sustenance is being supplanted by a more nuanced comprehension of individual fluctuation. Hereditary elements, specifically, assume a urgent part in molding how our bodies answer different dietary examples. The field of customized nourishment, utilizing hereditary data to tailor dietary suggestions, holds guarantee in giving more exact and compelling direction.

The Mediterranean eating routine stands apart as an immortal illustration of a dietary example that has gone the distance. Established in the conventional dietary patterns of nations lining the Mediterranean Ocean, this diet is described by a high admission of natural products, vegetables, entire grains, and olive oil, with moderate utilization of fish, poultry, and dairy.

Various investigations have connected the Mediterranean eating regimen to a lower hazard of coronary illness, stroke, and other constant circumstances.

What separates the Mediterranean eating routine is its all encompassing methodology. Instead of focusing on unambiguous supplements or nutrition types, it underlines the general dietary example and way of life factors. Normal actual work, social associations, and the delight in feasts are necessary parts of this methodology. The Mediterranean eating routine fills in as an update that the way to wellbeing might lie in the cooperative energy of different components as opposed to separated dietary decisions.

The idea of customized nourishment, while promising, is still in its early stages. How we might interpret the mind boggling interchange among hereditary qualities and nourishment is growing, yet useful applications for customized dietary proposals are not yet generally accessible. As this field develops, it can possibly alter how people approach their dietary decisions, creating some distance from conventional exhortation towards customized plans that think about individual hereditary cosmetics.

In the time of data, web-based entertainment stages assume a critical part in forming dietary patterns. Powerhouses, VIPs, and health masters utilize these stages to underwrite explicit eating regimens, adding to their quick scattering and reception. While virtual entertainment can be an important wellspring of data, moving toward dietary suggestions with a basic eye is fundamental. Narrative examples of overcoming adversity and sensationalized cases ought to be investigated against the background of logical proof and individual requirements.

The idea of "clean eating" has built up momentum lately, determined by a craving for natural, healthy food varieties. Clean eating energizes the utilization of entire, supplement thick food sources while staying away from or limiting handled and refined choices. While the goal behind clean eating is estimable, it can in some cases lead to prohibitive ways of behaving and an excessively unbending way to deal with food decisions.

Orthorexia nervosa, a term begat to depict a fixation on smart dieting, embodies the expected traps of taking clean eating to a limit. People with orthorexia may become focused on the virtue of their food decisions, prompting uneasiness and social seclusion. Adjusting the quest for nutritious food sources with an adaptable and pleasant way to deal with eating is urgent for keeping a solid relationship with food.

The impact of the food business on dietary patterns couldn't possibly be more significant. Promoting methodologies, item marking, and the accessibility of handled food sources shape shopper decisions in significant ways. Terms like "superfood" and "utilitarian food sources" are many times used to advertise explicit items as having remarkable medical advantages. While certain food varieties are to be sure supplement thick and deal wellbeing advancing properties, moving toward such cases with a basic eye is critical.

Financial factors likewise assume a huge part in deciding dietary examples. Admittance to new, nutritious food sources might be restricted in specific networks, prompting differences in wellbeing results. The expense of natural or specialty items, frequently connected with wellbeing centered counts calories, may present difficulties for people with lower livelihoods. Tending to these imbalances requires a thorough methodology, including strategy changes, local area drives, and training on reasonable and nutritious food decisions.

The idea of careful eating offers an offset to the high speed, diverted dietary patterns predominant in current culture. Careful eating includes focusing on the tactile parts of eating, like taste, surface, and smell, while monitoring craving and completion signs. This approach empowers a more deliberate and pleasant relationship with food, encouraging a more prominent appreciation for the eating experience.

Social variety essentially impacts dietary inclinations and practices. Conventional eating regimens, went down through ages, frequently reflect social qualities, strict convictions, and culinary practices. Investigating and commending the variety of worldwide cooking styles can expand one's sense of taste and add to a more comprehensive comprehension of sustenance.

The natural effect of food decisions has turned into a point of convergence in late conversations about feasible living. The carbon impression of various dietary examples, especially the creation of creature items, has prompted expanded interest in reasonable eating. A few people decide to diminish their meat utilization or settle on plant-based options as a method for reducing their natural effect. Notwithstanding, it is fundamental to think about the more extensive picture, including the ecological effect of plant agribusiness and transportation.

The interconnection among nourishment and emotional wellness is an arising area of examination. The stomach cerebrum hub, a bidirectional correspondence network connecting the gastrointestinal framework with the focal sensory system, is a central participant in this relationship. Certain dietary examples, like the Mediterranean eating routine, have been related with a lower hazard of sadness and mental degradation.

Then again, psychological wellness conditions can impact dietary decisions, frequently prompting profound or stress-related eating. Understanding the exchange among sustenance and psychological well-being has suggestions for both preventive and restorative intercessions. Integrating psychological well-being contemplations into conversations about dietary patterns is significant for advancing comprehensive prosperity.

As people explore the labyrinth of dietary patterns, encouraging a feeling of independence and self-empathy is central. The strain to adjust to a specific eating regimen or accomplish a particular self-perception can add to disarranged eating designs and adversely influence emotional well-being.

A more comprehensive and merciful way to deal with wellbeing and sustenance perceives that prosperity is diverse and can't be diminished to a bunch of inflexible principles.

All in all, the examination of well known dietary patterns uncovers a complicated exchange of likely advantages and downsides. Plant-based eating, irregular fasting, the ketogenic diet, and different patterns offer extraordinary benefits, however their viability relies upon individual elements and contemplations. Customized nourishment, the Mediterranean eating regimen, and careful eating give elective systems that focus on a comprehensive way to deal with wellbeing.

The impact of online entertainment, the food business, financial elements, and social variety highlights the diverse idea of dietary patterns. As people explore through this unpredictable scene, decisive reasoning and a familiarity with individual necessities are fundamental. Accomplishing a harmony between proof based suggestions and individual inclinations can prompt a feasible and satisfying way to deal with sustenance.

The excursion through dietary patterns is progressing, set apart by consistent movements and disclosures. Remaining receptive, embracing variety, and keeping a nuanced comprehension of sustenance will enable people to pursue informed decisions that line up with their qualities and add to their general prosperity.

5.2 Offering guidance on how to critically evaluate diet fads and choose a sustainable and balanced approach to nutrition.

In reality as we know it where data about sustenance is promptly accessible and continually developing, exploring the domain of diet patterns can be an overwhelming undertaking. From the most recent crazes elevated by famous people to old methods of reasoning rediscovered, people are besieged with changed and now and again clashing counsel on the most proficient method to eat for ideal wellbeing. The test lies in recognizing proof based proposals and sensationalized claims, eventually choosing a methodology that isn't just powerful yet additionally supportable over the long haul.

One of the essential standards in basically assessing diet patterns is grasping the logical premise behind the proposals. Thorough logical exploration is the best quality level for laying out the legitimacy of dietary mediations. As you experience another eating regimen pattern, dig into the accessible writing to distinguish peer-inspected examinations supporting or discrediting its cases. Be careful of narrative proof and be careful about proposals dependent exclusively upon individual encounters or tributes.

Consider the wellspring of data while assessing an eating routine pattern. Respectable logical diaries, wellbeing associations, and enlisted dietitians are solid hotspots for proof based data. Nonetheless, the ascent of virtual entertainment has presented a plenty of powerhouses, bloggers, and self-broadcasted nourishment specialists sharing their viewpoints.

While a portion of these people might give important experiences, it is pivotal to basically survey their capabilities, the exactness of their data, and whether their proposals line up with laid out dietary rules.

While investigating an eating regimen pattern, inspecting the broadness and profundity of the accessible research is fundamental. A solitary report, regardless of how promising, may not give a far reaching comprehension of the eating routine's effect on wellbeing. Search for a collection of proof comprising of numerous investigations, including randomized controlled preliminaries, efficient surveys, and meta-examinations. Predictable discoveries across various kinds of exploration add to the strength of the proof.

Assess the procedure of the examinations supporting an eating routine pattern. Consider factors, for example, test size, concentrate on length, and the measurable techniques utilized. Huge, all around planned investigations led over a lengthy period are by and large more dependable than little, momentary examinations with restrictions. Also, be careful of singled out information or studies that don't represent puzzling factors.

Understanding the potential predispositions innate in research is essential while fundamentally surveying diet patterns. Monetary irreconcilable circumstances, industry sponsorship, and scientist predisposition can impact concentrate on results. Assess whether the scientists have unveiled any likely irreconcilable circumstances and consider what these variables might mean for the understanding of the outcomes. Free examinations not subsidized by industry sources are by and large more reliable.

While logical proof structures the establishment for assessing diet patterns, taking into account individual variability is similarly significant. Bodies answer diversely to different dietary methodologies because of variables like hereditary qualities, age, orientation, and basic ailments. Perceive that what works for one individual may not be reasonable for another. Survey your own wellbeing status, dietary inclinations, and way of life while considering a specific eating regimen pattern to guarantee it lines up with your singular necessities.

Chasing ideal wellbeing, it's pivotal to take on a comprehensive perspective on nourishment that includes what you eat as well as how you eat. As opposed to focusing on unambiguous supplements or superfoods, center around developing a fair and differed diet. An eating regimen wealthy in different natural products, vegetables, entire grains, lean proteins, and solid fats gives an expansive range of fundamental supplements. Go for the gold plate that mirrors the variety of supplement rich food varieties accessible.

Notwithstanding food decisions, focusing on segment sizes and careful eating rehearses adds to a reasonable methodology. Pay attention to your body's appetite and completion signs, enjoy the kinds of your feasts, and keep away from interruptions during eating.

Consolidate different cooking strategies and culinary methods to upgrade the delight in your dinners, encouraging a positive relationship with food.

The significance of supportability in dietary decisions reaches out past the environmental sense to envelop long haul adherence to a picked eating design. While some eating routine patterns might yield quick outcomes for the time being, their supportability over a drawn out period is a basic thought. Consumes less calories that are excessively prohibitive, killing whole nutritional categories or depending on unreasonable eating plans, might be trying to keep up with over the long haul.

Survey the reasonableness and possibility of an eating regimen pattern inside the setting of your day to day routine. Consider whether the suggested food sources are promptly accessible, reasonable, and line up with your social inclinations. Assess how well the eating regimen squeezes into your public activity, work responsibilities, and in general way of life. A reasonable way to deal with sustenance is one that flawlessly coordinates with your everyday practice and takes into consideration adaptability and happiness.

One more key part of assessing diet patterns is analyzing their possible effect on psychological wellness. Outrageous dietary limitations or a consistent spotlight on "clean" eating can add to the improvement of disarranged eating designs. Orthorexia nervosa, described by a fanatical obsession with good dieting, is an illustration of what an excessively inflexible way to deal with nourishment can adversely mean for mental prosperity. Focus on a fair and adaptable mentality towards food to keep a positive relationship with eating.

Understanding the job of social impacts in molding dietary decisions is funda-mental for an exhaustive assessment of diet patterns. Conventional weight control plans, frequently went down through ages, reflect social qualities, culinary customs, and neighborhood fixings. Perceive that social variety adds to the wealth of worldwide cooking and that there is nobody size-fits-all way to deal with nourishment. Embrace the potential chance to investigate and commend the range of food varieties from various societies, coordinating them into a reasonable and comprehensive dietary example.

In the ongoing period of data over-burden, online entertainment assumes a critical part in the scattering of diet patterns. While it tends to be an important wellspring of motivation and backing, it likewise presents difficulties regarding deception and the advancement of unreasonable body goals. While experiencing diet patterns via web-based entertainment, fundamentally assess the accreditations of the people or associations sharing the data. Consider whether the suggestions line up with laid out healthful rules and whether they depend on logical proof.

Be aware of the potential for social examination and the impact of unreasonable body norms pervasive via virtual entertainment stages. Perceive that organized pictures and examples of overcoming adversity may not give an extensive image of the diffi-culties and intricacies people face in executing explicit eating routine patterns. Center around your own wellbeing objectives, progress, and prosperity, as opposed to taking a stab at a romanticized picture advanced in web-based spaces.

The food business' part in forming dietary patterns can't be disregarded. The adver-tising of items as "superfoods" or "wonder arrangements" can add to the notoriety of explicit dietary methodologies. While assessing diet patterns, know about the impact of showcasing techniques, item marking, and the commodification of wellbeing. Con-sider whether the proposals line up with a decent and proof based way to deal with nourishment or on the other hand on the off chance that they are basically determined by business interests.

Financial elements assume an essential part in deciding admittance to and moder-ateness of specific food sources, impacting dietary examples. Perceive that people with changing pay levels might confront various difficulties in getting to new, nutritious food varieties. Tending to food imbalances requires a more extensive cultural methodology, including strategy changes, local area drives, and training on reasonable and quality food decisions.

A fundamental part of a reasonable way to deal with nourishment is recognizing the interconnectedness of physical and mental prosperity. Arising research features the bidirectional connection among diet and emotional well-being. Certain dietary examples, like the Mediterranean eating regimen, have been related with a lower chance of wretchedness and mental deterioration. On the other hand, emotional wellness conditions can impact eating ways of behaving, highlighting the significance of thinking about the two viewpoints for generally speaking prosperity.

While assessing diet patterns, it is vital to perceive that wellbeing is diverse and can't be decreased to a bunch of inflexible guidelines. A customized way to deal with sustenance, considering individual necessities, inclinations, and wellbeing objectives, is critical to accomplishing economical and long haul achievement. Meeting with medical care experts, including enrolled dietitians, can give customized direction in light of your exceptional wellbeing profile.

All in all, offering direction on fundamentally assessing diet trends and picking a reasonable and adjusted way to deal with sustenance requires a multi-layered approach. Understanding the logical premise of diet patterns, taking into account individual inconstancy, embracing an all encompassing perspective on sustenance, and focusing on manageability and mental prosperity are fundamental parts of this interaction.

As people explore the mind boggling scene of dietary decisions, engaging them with the instruments to settle on informed choices guarantees a way to ideal wellbeing that is proof based, sensible, and helpful for long haul prosperity.

In the steadily developing scene of nourishment, the mission for a practical and adjusted approach is of principal significance. In the midst of the horde of dietary patterns, trends, and clashing counsel, people look for direction on the most proficient method to feed their bodies in a manner that advances wellbeing, life span, and by and large prosperity. This excursion towards a feasible and adjusted approach includes basic assessment, a comprehension of individual necessities, and an all encompassing point of view that reaches out past simple food decisions.

At the center of picking a manageable and adjusted way to deal with sustenance is the basic assessment of dietary patterns. During a time where data is effectively open, people are immersed with different weight control plans promising convenient solutions and extraordinary results. From plant-based eating to irregular fasting, each pattern accompanies its own arrangement of cases and suggestions. To explore this complex scene, it is vital to apply an insightful eye, isolating proof based guidance from sensationalized claims.

Logical proficiency assumes a crucial part in this basic assessment process. Understanding the technique of exploration studies, knowing among connection and causation, and deciphering measurable importance are fundamental abilities. While evaluating the legitimacy of a dietary pattern, it is basic to dig into the logical writing, looking for peer-inspected investigations and meta-examinations that give an extensive outline of the accessible proof. A dependence on thorough examination shapes the establishment for coming to informed and proof based conclusions about dietary decisions.

Thought of the wellspring of data is similarly essential in the mission for a fair way to deal with sustenance. Legitimate sources, for example, peer-checked on diaries, wellbeing associations, and enlisted dietitians give dependable and proof based data. Interestingly, the ascent of web-based entertainment has given a stage to forces to be reckoned with, bloggers, and self-declared nourishment specialists. While these people might offer important bits of knowledge, it is fundamental to examine their capabilities, evaluate the precision of their data, and question whether their proposals line up with laid out wholesome rules.

As people explore the ocean of dietary patterns, understanding the subtleties of logical exploration becomes significant. The broadness and profundity of accessible proof add to the dependability of a given dietary pattern. Various all around planned investigations, including randomized controlled preliminaries and efficient audits, improve the vigor of the proof. Steady discoveries across different exploration strategies loan validity to the possible advantages or downsides related with a specific dietary methodology.

One more aspect of basic assessment includes thinking about potential predispositions inborn in research. Monetary irreconcilable circumstances, industry sponsorship, and specialist predisposition can impact concentrate on results and translations. Inspecting whether analysts have uncovered irreconcilable circumstances and evaluating the autonomy of subsidizing sources upgrades the capacity to recognize the dependability of the discoveries. Consciousness of potential inclinations is necessary to coming to informed conclusions about dietary decisions.

While logical proof structures the foundation of a fair way to deal with sustenance, it is similarly vital to perceive individual fluctuation. Bodies answer diversely to different dietary examples because of elements like hereditary qualities, age, orientation, and basic ailments. The affirmation that what works for one individual may not be reasonable for one more stresses the significance of fitting dietary decisions to individual necessities.

Personalization reaches out past hereditary variables to envelop way of life, inclinations, and social contemplations. A feasible and adjusted way to deal with sustenance considers the healthful requirements of the person as well as the common sense of integrating these decisions into day to day existence. This customized point of view cultivates a more comprehensive and versatile way to deal with sustenance that lines up with individual inclinations and real factors.

The comprehensive perspective on nourishment includes perceiving that food isn't just fuel; it is a wellspring of delight, culture, and social association. Embracing a reasonable methodology involves valuing the different exhibit of food varieties accessible and developing a positive relationship with eating. Instead of focusing on unambiguous supplements or belittling specific food varieties, the emphasis is on feeding the body while getting joy and fulfillment from the eating experience.

A reasonable eating routine, described by assortment and balance, is fundamental to a maintainable way to deal with sustenance. The incorporation of a different scope of food sources guarantees the admission of fundamental supplements, nutrients, and minerals important for ideal wellbeing. Organic products, vegetables, entire grains, lean proteins, and sound fats comprise the structure blocks of a balanced and healthfully complete eating regimen.

Understanding part estimates and rehearsing careful eating are essential parts of a decent methodology. Careful eating includes being available during feasts, focusing on appetite and totality signs, and appreciating the kinds of each nibble. This careful methodology cultivates a more prominent association with food and advances a sound connection with eating, lessening the probability of overconsumption or dependence on outer signals.

Manageability with regards to nourishment stretches out past biological contemplations to the drawn out adherence to a picked eating design.

While specific eating regimen patterns might yield quick outcomes at first, their maintainability over a lengthy period is a basic element. Consumes less calories that are excessively prohibitive, disposing of whole nutrition types or forcing unfeasible eating plans, might be trying to keep up with over the long haul.

Reasonableness and possibility are fundamental contemplations while assessing the manageability of a dietary methodology. Survey whether the suggested food varieties are promptly accessible, reasonable, and line up with social or individual inclinations. A maintainable eating regimen flawlessly incorporates into day to day existence, considering adaptability and flexibility to different circumstances. This versatility is urgent for exploring get-togethers, travel, and other genuine situations without compromising by and large dietary examples.

Social impacts assume a critical part in molding dietary decisions and inclinations. Customary eating regimens, frequently went down through ages, reflect social qualities, culinary practices, and nearby fixings. Perceiving and celebrating social variety add to a more comprehensive comprehension of sustenance. Embracing the extravagance of worldwide cooking styles and integrating different food sources into a reasonable eating routine changes it up and delight to the eating experience.

The effect of virtual entertainment on dietary decisions is unquestionable in the contemporary scene. Online entertainment stages act as channels for the scattering of dietary patterns, with powerhouses and superstars frequently supporting explicit methodologies. While web-based entertainment can be an important wellspring of motivation and backing, moving toward dietary proposals with an insightful eye is fundamental. Tales and examples of overcoming adversity ought to be examined against the background of logical proof and individual requirements.

The idea of "clean eating" has acquired ubiquity as of late, determined by a longing for natural, healthy food sources. While the aim behind clean eating is praiseworthy, it is critical to find some kind of harmony between focusing on supplement thick food sources and keeping an adaptable and charming way to deal with eating. An excessively unbending translation of clean eating can prompt prohibitive ways of behaving and possibly add to disarranged eating designs.

The impact of the food business on dietary decisions is one more variable to consider. Advertising procedures, item naming, and the accessibility of handled food varieties can shape buyer choices. Terms like "superfood" and "practical food sources" are much of the time used to advertise explicit items as having phenomenal medical advantages. While certain food varieties may for sure offer wellbeing advancing properties, it is crucial for approach such cases with a basic eye and think about the general dietary example.

Financial variables add to variations in dietary examples and admittance to nutritious food varieties. People with fluctuating pay levels might confront various difficulties in getting new, top notch food varieties. Tending to these imbalances requires a complex methodology, including strategy changes, local area drives, and training on reasonable and good food decisions. A decent way to deal with sustenance recognizes these financial factors and backers for impartial admittance to nutritious food varieties for all.

The interconnection among sustenance and emotional wellness is an arising area of examination. Certain dietary examples, like the Mediterranean eating regimen, have been related with a lower hazard of misery and mental degradation. On the other hand, psychological wellness conditions can impact eating ways of behaving, underscoring the bidirectional connection between the two. Perceiving the job of sustenance in mental prosperity adds a vital aspect to the idea of a reasonable way to deal with wellbeing.

Chapter 6

Mindful Eating Practices

Careful eating is a training that empowers an uplifted consciousness of the food we eat, our dietary patterns, and the sensations related with eating. It is established in the standards of care, which include focusing on the current second without judgment. With regards to eating, care permits people to foster a more profound association with their food, relish the flavors, and encourage a more certain relationship with eating.

One key part of careful eating is the development of mindfulness during dinners. This includes being completely present and taken part in the demonstration of eating, as opposed to devouring food in a careless, programmed way. In our high speed present day culture, it is normal for individuals to eat rapidly, perform various tasks during feasts, or eat in a hurry. Careful consuming empowers a shift from these propensities, advancing a more purposeful and cognizant way to deal with sustenance.

At the point when we eat carefully, we become sensitive to our body's appetite and completion signals. This includes paying attention to our body and eating when we are eager, halting when we are fulfilled, and perceiving the signs that show genuine actual craving versus close to home or fatigue driven eating. By fostering this mindfulness, people can cultivate a better relationship with food and abstain from gorging or undereating in view of outside signals.

Careful eating likewise accentuates the significance of relishing each nibble and valuing the tactile experience of eating. This incorporates focusing on the tones, surfaces, and kinds of the food, as well as the demonstration of biting and gulping. By completely captivating with the tactile parts of eating, people can get additional fulfillment from their dinners and decrease the propensity to overconsume trying to make up for an apparent shortfall.

Developing appreciation for the food we eat is one more key part of careful eating. Requiring a second to recognize the work and assets that went into creating the food on our plate can encourage a more noteworthy feeling of appreciation and association with the sustenance it gives. This part of care energizes a shift away from a conditional perspective on food utilization and towards a more significant comprehension of the interconnectedness of food creation, dissemination, and our own prosperity.

Notwithstanding the actual parts of eating, careful eating tends to the close to home and mental parts of our relationship with food. Many individuals use food as a method for adapting to pressure, tension, fatigue, or different feelings.

Careful eating urges people to investigate the close to home triggers behind their dietary patterns and foster other option, better strategies for dealing with especially difficult times. This mindfulness can prompt a more adjusted and economical way to deal with profound prosperity.

Careful eating is definitely not a one-size-fits-all training; rather, it very well may be custom fitted to individual inclinations and requirements. There are different methods and procedures that people can integrate into their regular routines to cultivate careful dietary patterns. One such strategy is the act of careful breathing before feasts. Taking a couple of profound, purposeful breaths assists with focusing the psyche, make a feeling of quiet, and lay out a careful presence prior to starting to eat.

Another powerful technique is to eat without interruptions, like switching off the TV, taking care of electronic gadgets, and zeroing in exclusively on the demonstration of eating. This permits people to completely draw in with their food and the eating system, lessening the probability of gorging and advancing a really fulfilling dinner experience.

Careful eating likewise includes focusing on yearning and completion signals all through a feast. This implies enjoying reprieves during eating to evaluate one's degree of completion and choosing whether to keep eating or stop. By integrating these stops, people can stay away from thoughtless indulging and better adjust themselves to their body's normal signs.

Biting food gradually and completely is a basic yet strong careful eating practice. This takes into consideration a more prominent enthusiasm for the flavors and surfaces of the food, as well as further developed processing. Eating gradually additionally gives the cerebrum additional opportunity to enlist signs of completion, decreasing the probability of overconsumption.

Segment control is one more significant part of careful eating. Being aware of piece sizes assists people with keeping away from exorbitant calorie consumption and urges a reasonable way to deal with nourishment. Utilizing more modest plates, serving sizes, and focusing on inward yearning and completion signals can add to a better relationship with food.

Careful eating stretches out past the demonstration of eating itself; it incorporates the whole food experience, from shopping and feast arrangement to the second the food is devoured. Being careful during shopping for food includes pursuing cognizant and nutritious decisions, choosing various entire food varieties, and monitoring the natural effect of food decisions.

Feast planning is an amazing chance to participate in careful exercises, for example, hacking vegetables, estimating fixings, and valuing the varieties and fragrances of the food being ready. This purposeful way to deal with feast arrangement can improve the general happiness and fulfillment got from the eating experience.

It's critical to take note of that careful eating isn't tied in with complying with severe standards or limitations. All things considered, it empowers adaptability and self-empathy. Permitting oneself to appreciate liberal food varieties with some restraint without culpability or judgment is predictable with the standards of careful eating. This approach assists people foster a reasonable and practical relationship with food, advancing both physical and mental prosperity.

Careful eating is especially useful for people looking to work on their general well-being and prosperity. Research recommends that careful eating practices can add to weight the executives, better processing, and worked on metabolic wellbeing. By encouraging a more certain and deliberate relationship with food, people might encounter upgraded fulfillment with dinners, diminished profound eating, and expanded in general life fulfillment.

Notwithstanding its actual medical advantages, careful eating has been related with upgrades in emotional well-being. For people battling with disarranged eating designs, for example, gorging or profound eating, careful eating can offer an important instrument for fostering a better relationship with food. The training energizes self-reflection and mindfulness, enabling people to pursue more cognizant decisions about their eating ways of behaving.

Careful eating has likewise been investigated as a reciprocal methodology in the treatment of different dietary problems, for example, anorexia nervosa, bulimia nervosa, and gorging jumble. While it's anything but an independent treatment, integrating careful eating standards into an exhaustive remedial arrangement can uphold people in fostering a more offset and maintainable relationship with food.

The utilization of careful eating reaches out to different settings, including instructive foundations, work environments, and local area programs. Incorporating careful eating rehearses into school educational programs can assist youngsters with creating smart dieting propensities and a positive relationship with food since the beginning. Additionally, working environments can advance careful eating by establishing steady conditions, for example, assigned eating spaces liberated from interruptions.

Local area programs that integrate careful eating studios or occasions can give significant assets and backing to people looking to embrace better dietary patterns. These drives can encourage a feeling of local area and shared obligation to careful living.

Developing careful eating rehearses requires continuous exertion and responsibility. Similarly as with any propensity or expertise, integrating care into dietary patterns might take time and practice. It's fundamental for approach the interaction with persistence, self-empathy, and a readiness to gain from the two triumphs and difficulties.

Careful eating is definitely not an unbending arrangement of rules but instead an adaptable and individualized way to deal with supporting the body and psyche. As people set out on their careful eating venture, they might find special methodologies and procedures that impact them by and by. The key is to stay open to trial and error and transformation, permitting the training to develop and turn into a manageable piece of one's way of life.

All in all, careful eating is an all encompassing and deliberate way to deal with sustenance that goes past the demonstration of devouring food. It includes developing mindfulness, appreciation, and appreciation for the whole food experience, from choice and arrangement to utilization. By cultivating a careful relationship with food, people can upgrade their general prosperity, work on their psychological and close to home association with eating, and advance a better way of life. The standards of careful eating offer an important structure for creating maintainable and positive dietary patterns that add to long haul wellbeing and essentialness.

6.1 Introducing the concept of mindful eating and its impact on overall health.

Presenting the idea of careful gobbling opens up a groundbreaking point of view on our relationship with food and its effect on generally wellbeing. Careful eating is a training well established in the standards of care, which includes developing an intense consciousness of the current second without judgment. When applied to eating, this care urges people to move toward their dinners with aim, consideration, and an increased feeling of mindfulness. The ramifications of embracing careful eating reach out a long ways past the demonstration of devouring food; they envelop physical, mental, and close to home prosperity.

Amidst our speedy and frequently rushed lives, a considerable lot of us have created propensities for thoughtless eating. This includes consuming dinners absent a lot of thought, frequently in a rushed or diverted way. Careful eating, conversely, prompts us to dial back and really experience the most common way of sustaining our bodies. It energizes a shift away from autopilot eating, permitting us to enjoy the flavors, surfaces, and by and large tangible experience of our dinners.

At its center, careful eating underlines the significance of being available during feasts. This includes dismissing our consideration from outside interruptions, for example, cell phones or TV, and completely captivating with the demonstration of eating. By carrying attention to the current second, people can reconnect with their bodies and the signs they give in regards to appetite and completion. This uplifted mindfulness makes way for a more adjusted and careful way to deal with sustenance.

One crucial part of careful eating is the development of a cognizant familiarity with craving and totality prompts. In the rushing about of day to day existence, it's normal for people to eat in view of outside prompts, like season of day or social impacts, as opposed to paying attention to their body's regular signs.

Careful eating urges people to become sensitive to their actual sensations, recognizing genuine yearning and close to home or ongoing eating. This mindfulness can be an integral asset in advancing a better relationship with food and forestalling gorging.

In the excursion of careful eating, the idea of "eating with goal" arises as a key guideline. It includes settling on conscious decisions about what to eat, for what reason to eat, and how to eat. Purposeful eating welcomes people to think about the healthy benefit of their food, their own inclinations, and the effect of their decisions on their general prosperity. By moving toward feasts with expectation, people can encourage a feeling of strengthening and play a functioning job in forming their dietary propensities.

Careful eating additionally focuses on the profound and mental parts of our relationship with food. Numerous people go to food as a wellspring of solace, stress help, or a method for adapting to feelings. Careful eating urges people to investigate the close to home triggers behind their dietary patterns, encouraging a more profound comprehension of the association among feelings and food. This self-reflection can be a urgent move toward creating better survival strategies and breaking liberated from examples of close to home eating.

One of the vital practices in careful eating includes relishing each chomp. This goes past only devouring nourishment for food; it includes valuing the tactile experience of eating. By focusing on the tones, surfaces, and kinds of the food, people can get more prominent fulfillment from their feasts. The purposeful demonstration of biting and relishing each nibble improves the happiness regarding the feast as well as permits the body to enlist satiety all the more successfully, diminishing the probability of indulging.

Appreciation turns into a focal subject in the careful eating venture. Offering thanks for the food we eat includes perceiving the work and assets that went into delivering the dinner. Whether the ranchers developed the produce, the hands that pre-arranged the dinner, or the Earth that gave the fixings, recognizing this interconnected trap of connections adds a significant aspect to the demonstration of eating. Appreciation encourages a feeling of appreciation and care, supporting that eating isn't simply a value-based process however an all encompassing encounter.

The act of careful breathing is frequently entwined with careful eating. Taking a couple of seconds to participate in profound, deliberate breaths before a dinner effectively focuses the brain and make a feeling of quiet. This careful presence laid out through breathing assists people with changing from the requests of day to day existence to the supporting demonstration of eating. It establishes the vibe for a more deliberate and cognizant way to deal with the dinner, making space for appreciation and mindfulness.

Careful eating isn't about prohibitive weight control plans or inflexible guidelines; rather, it empowers an adaptable and humane mentality towards oneself.

Considering the delight in liberal food varieties with some restraint, without culpability or judgment, lines up with the standards of careful eating. This non-prohibitive methodology advances a better relationship with food, underlining equilibrium and care over hardship.

As people set out on the excursion of careful eating, they frequently track down esteem in the act of eating without interruptions. This includes making a committed reality for feasts, liberated from the interruption of electronic gadgets or different interruptions. By zeroing in exclusively on the demonstration of eating, people can completely draw in with their food and the eating system, prompting a really fulfilling and careful feast insight.

Biting food gradually and completely is a basic yet significant careful eating practice. This conscious methodology permits people to completely see the value in the surfaces and kinds of the food, while likewise advancing better absorption. Eating gradually gives the cerebrum additional opportunity to enlist signs of completion, lessening the probability of overconsumption. This act of careful biting lines up with the general topic of dialing back and being available during feasts.

Segment control is one more fundamental part of careful eating. Focusing on segment sizes assists people with staying away from extreme calorie consumption and elevates a decent way to deal with sustenance. Careful piece control includes utilizing more modest plates, being aware of serving sizes, and being sensitive to interior yearning and completion prompts. This training adds to a better relationship with food, underscoring higher expectations no matter what.

Careful eating reaches out past the demonstration of eating itself; it envelops the whole food experience, from the determination of fixings to feast arrangement. Careful shopping for food includes settling on deliberate and nutritious decisions, choosing different entire food sources, and monitoring the natural effect of food decisions. This care in choosing fixings sets the establishment for a feeding and reasonable eating experience.

Feast readiness turns into a chance for careful commitment with the food we eat. Exercises, for example, cleaving vegetables, estimating fixings, and valuing the varieties and fragrances of the food add to the generally careful eating experience. This purposeful way to deal with dinner readiness upgrades the fulfillment got from the eating system and builds up the interconnectedness of each move toward the food venture.

The standards of careful eating can be applied to different settings, including instructive organizations, working environments, and local area programs. Integrating careful eating into school educational programs can assume a pivotal part in forming the dietary patterns of youthful people. By giving instruction and down to earth devices to careful eating, schools can enable understudies to settle on better decisions and foster a positive relationship with food since the beginning.

Work environments can add to the advancement of careful eating by establishing steady conditions. This might include laying out assigned eating spaces liberated from interruptions, empowering workers to enjoy careful reprieves during feasts, and giving instructive assets on the advantages of careful eating. Such work environment drives can cultivate a culture of prosperity and care, decidedly influencing the wellbeing and efficiency of representatives.

Local area programs that incorporate careful eating studios or occasions offer significant assets for people trying to take on better dietary patterns. These projects give a steady space to sharing encounters, learning careful eating strategies, and building a feeling of local area around careful living. By expanding the act of careful eating to the local area level, these projects add to an aggregate obligation to better and more careful living.

Developing careful eating rehearses requires continuous exertion and responsibility. Like any propensity or expertise, integrating care into dietary patterns might take time and practice. It's crucial for approach the interaction with persistence, self-empathy, and a readiness to gain from the two triumphs and difficulties.

As people dive into the act of careful eating, they might find novel procedures and strategies that impact them by and by. The key is to stay open to trial and error and transformation, permitting the training to develop and turn into a feasible piece of one's way of life. Careful eating is certainly not an inflexible arrangement of rules yet rather an adaptable and individualized way to deal with sustaining the body and brain.

Research demonstrates that careful eating practices can add to different parts of wellbeing and prosperity. Weight the board is one region where careful eating makes shown positive impacts. By advancing a more purposeful and mindful way to deal with eating, people might turn out to be more sensitive to their body's signs of craving and completion, prompting better weight control.

Further developed assimilation is one more likely advantage of careful eating. The act of biting food completely and enjoying each nibble can upgrade the stomach related process, permitting the body to extricate greatest supplements from the food devoured. This might add to better generally speaking stomach related wellbeing and supplement retention.

Metabolic wellbeing is a key viewpoint impacted by careful eating rehearses. By encouraging a more adjusted and careful way to deal with food decisions, people might encounter enhancements in metabolic markers, for example, glucose levels and insulin responsiveness. These positive changes add to a diminished gamble of metabolic problems and backing generally speaking metabolic prosperity.

The emotional wellness advantages of careful eating are critical. For people battling with confused eating designs, for example, pigging out or close to home eating, careful eating can offer a significant instrument for fostering a better relationship with food. The training supports self-reflection and mindfulness, enabling people to pursue more cognizant decisions about their eating ways of behaving.

Besides, careful eating has been investigated as a reciprocal methodology in the treatment of different dietary problems, including anorexia nervosa, bulimia nervosa, and voraciously consuming food issue. While it's anything but an independent treatment, integrating careful eating standards into a complete remedial arrangement can uphold people in fostering a more offset and maintainable relationship with food.

The advantages of careful eating reach out past the singular level to influence cultural prosperity. As additional people embrace careful eating rehearses, there is potential for positive changes in dietary propensities, food decisions, and in general wellbeing results for a bigger scope. This aggregate obligation to care in eating adds to a culture of prosperity and better living.

All in all, presenting the idea of careful eating is an encouragement to change our relationship with food and, likewise, our general wellbeing. Careful eating is definitely not a prohibitive eating routine or a bunch of inflexible principles; rather, it is an all encompassing and deliberate way to deal with sustenance. By developing mindfulness, appreciation, and appreciation for the whole food experience, people can improve their prosperity, both genuinely and intellectually.

The act of careful eating urges people to be available during dinners, pay attention to their body's signs, and move toward eating with goal. It includes enjoying each chomp, offering thanks for the food ate, and perceiving the close to home and mental parts of eating. Careful eating is an excursion that reaches out from the determination of fixings to the readiness and utilization of dinners, advancing a feeling of interconnectedness with the food we eat.

As people set out on the careful eating venture, they find the force of purposeful decisions, the delight of appreciating each experience, and the significant effect on their general wellbeing. Careful eating is an adaptable and individualized work on, requiring progressing responsibility and an eagerness to embrace a more cognizant way to deal with feeding the body and brain. In the journey for a better and more careful life, the standards of careful eating give an important aide, cultivating an agreeable relationship with food and advancing enduring prosperity.

6.2 Techniques for cultivating awareness during meals to enhance digestion and promote better food choices.

Developing mindfulness during dinners is a crucial part of careful eating that can significantly affect processing and advance better food decisions. In our high speed, present day lives, it's not difficult to fall into the propensity for eating rapidly and absent a lot of thought. This thoughtless way to deal with feasts can add to unfortunate processing, gorging, and a separation from the tangible experience of eating. By integrating explicit strategies to improve mindfulness during feasts, people can encourage a more deliberate and careful relationship with their food.

One method for developing mindfulness during feasts is in the first place a snapshot of careful relaxing. Prior to taking the primary nibble, people can take a couple of full breaths to focus themselves and carry their regard for the current second. This basic practice makes a psychological shift from the rushing about of day to day existence to the feeding demonstration of eating. Careful breathing makes way for a more deliberate and cognizant way to deal with the dinner, making an establishment for uplifted mindfulness.

Biting food gradually and completely is a strong strategy for improving mindfulness during dinners. Numerous people are acquainted with racing through their dinners, taking enormous chomps, and gulping absent a lot of thought. By dialing back the biting system, people can completely draw in with the surfaces and kinds of their food. This conscious methodology not just advances better absorption by separating food all the more successfully yet in addition permits the mind to enroll satiety, lessening the probability of gorging.

One more procedure for developing mindfulness is to eat without interruptions. In the present innovation driven world, it's not unexpected to eat while staring at the TV, looking at virtual entertainment, or dealing with a PC. Nonetheless, these interruptions redirect consideration from the eating experience, making it trying to see the value in the flavors and surfaces of the food completely. By making a devoted existence for feasts without electronic gadgets or different interruptions, people can submerge themselves in the demonstration of eating, cultivating a more profound association with their food.

Careful part control is a method that includes being aware of serving sizes and focusing on inner craving and totality signs. As opposed to depending on outer signals or cultural assumptions, people can foster a more natural comprehension of how much food their body needs. This method urges a reasonable way to deal with nourishment and forestalls overconsumption, adding to better processing and generally prosperity.

Focusing on the varieties, surfaces, and kinds of the food is a tangible method that upgrades mindfulness during dinners. Frequently, people consume dinners without genuinely enjoying the tactile experience.

Careful eating includes connecting every one of the faculties, from the visual allure of the food on the plate to the fragrances and tastes experienced with each nibble. By effectively valuing the tangible parts of eating, people get more prominent fulfillment from their dinners and are less inclined to depend on outer signals for delight.

The act of careful eating includes recognizing and offering thanks for the food being devoured. Pausing for a minute to consider the work and assets that went into delivering the dinner encourages a feeling of appreciation. This appreciation stretches out past the singular demonstration of eating, perceiving the interconnected snare of connections engaged with offering food of real value. By integrating appreciation into feasts, people foster a more careful and positive relationship with their food, adding to a better generally speaking experience.

Careful eating additionally urges people to know about their body's appetite and completion prompts. This includes checking out the actual impressions that demonstrate genuine appetite and perceiving when the body has had enough to eat. By being sensitive to these signals, people can go with additional educated decisions about when to begin and quit eating, advancing a decent and instinctive way to deal with sustenance. This method upholds absorption by adjusting dietary patterns to the body's normal signs.

A method that lines up with careful eating is the idea of "eating with aim." This includes settling on conscious decisions about what to eat, for what reason to eat, and how to eat. By moving toward dinners with goal, people can think about the dietary benefit of their food, their own inclinations, and the effect of their decisions on their general prosperity. Eating with goal engages people to play a functioning job in forming their dietary propensities and cultivates a feeling of control and care.

Rehearsing careful eating likewise incorporates enjoying reprieves during feasts to evaluate one's degree of completion. This method includes stopping during the feast to ponder how eager or fulfilled one feels. By consolidating these breaks, people can stay away from thoughtless indulging and foster a more prominent familiarity with their body's signs. This strategy upholds absorption by permitting the stomach related framework time to actually process and sign completion.

Integrating careful eating rehearses into dinner planning is one more method for upgrading mindfulness during feasts. Exercises, for example, cleaving vegetables, estimating fixings, and valuing the varieties and smells of the food add to the generally careful eating experience. By participating in deliberate activities during dinner arrangement, people can convey that care into the eating system, building up the association between the food and the demonstration of feeding the body.

A method that empowers mindfulness and care is the idea of careful shopping for food. This includes settling on deliberate and nutritious decisions while choosing fixings. Being careful during shopping for food incorporates picking various entire food sources, monitoring dietary names, and taking into account the natural effect of food decisions. By moving toward shopping for food with care, people set up for a feeding and deliberate eating experience.

Establishing a steady eating climate is a strategy that adds to developing mindfulness during feasts. This includes picking a calm and agreeable space for feasts, liberated from interruptions and outside pressures. By establishing a quiet climate, people can zero in on the demonstration of eating, advancing a more careful and pleasant feast insight. This procedure upgrades assimilation by decreasing pressure and permitting the body to participate during the time spent sustenance completely.

Careful eating additionally urges people to investigate the profound and mental parts of their relationship with food. This strategy includes self-reflection on the close to home triggers behind dietary patterns. By acquiring understanding into the association among feelings and food decisions, people can arrive at additional cognizant conclusions about their eating ways of behaving. This mindfulness upholds better food decisions and a better generally relationship with food.

Taking part in careful eating rehearses stretches out past individual endeavors to cultural prosperity. By advancing mindfulness during dinners, there is the potential for positive changes in dietary propensities, food decisions, and generally speaking wellbeing results for a bigger scope. This aggregate obligation to care in eating adds to a culture of prosperity and better living at the local area level.

Taking everything into account, procedures for developing mindfulness during dinners are fundamental for upgrading processing and advancing better food decisions. These procedures, established in the standards of careful eating, urge people to dial back, enjoy each nibble, and completely draw in with the tangible experience of eating. By consolidating careful breathing, biting gradually, keeping away from interruptions, rehearsing segment control, and offering thanks, people can encourage a more deliberate and careful relationship with their food. These methods upgrade processing as well as add to by and large prosperity, supporting a better and more cognizant way to deal with sustenance.

6.3 Mindful eating exercises and practices.

Careful eating activities and practices assume a urgent part in encouraging a more profound association with food, advancing generally speaking prosperity, and developing a careful way to deal with sustenance. These activities are intended to carry attention to the current second, upgrade the tangible experience of eating, and support deliberate decisions. Integrating these practices into day to day existence can prompt a more offset and amicable relationship with food.

One central careful eating exercise includes careful breathing before feasts. This training fills in as an establishing strategy, permitting people to progress from the hecticness of day to day existence to the current snapshot of eating. Prior to taking the primary nibble, people can take a couple of full breaths, zeroing in on the inward breath and exhalation. This purposeful breathing makes a feeling of quiet and presence, making way for a more careful and deliberate way to deal with the feast.

One more remarkable careful eating exercise is the act of eating without interruptions. This includes making a committed eating space liberated from electronic gadgets, TV, or other outer interruptions. By eliminating these interruptions, people can completely submerge themselves in the demonstration of eating, carrying elevated attention to the flavors, surfaces, and in general tactile experience of the food. This exercise supports a more careful and purposeful relationship with dinners.

Biting carefully is a basic yet compelling activity that advances mindfulness during dinners. Rather than hurrying through nibbles, people can zero in on the demonstration of biting, focusing on the surfaces and kinds of the food. This conscious methodology improves the satisfaction in the dinner as well as supports better absorption. Careful biting permits people to enjoy each nibble, making a really fulfilling and careful eating experience.

The raisin practice is an exemplary care practice that can be adjusted to careful eating. In this activity, people take a couple of seconds to notice a raisin intently prior to eating it. They notice the variety, surface, and state of the raisin, and afterward continue to eat it gradually, relishing each nibble. This exercise empowers an elevated consciousness of the tangible parts of eating and can be applied to different food sources, encouraging a more profound association with the demonstration of sustaining the body.

Rehearsing appreciation before feasts is a careful eating exercise that includes communicating appreciation for the food being devoured. People can pause for a minute to consider the excursion of the food from its source to their plate, recognizing the work of those engaged with its creation. This exercise encourages a feeling of appreciation for the sustenance the food gives and advances a good and careful outlook prior to eating.

A careful eating exercise that spotlights on segment control is the "plate stop." This includes having some time off part of the way through the dinner to evaluate one's degree of completion. People can put down their utensils, pause for a minute to check in with their body, and choose whether to keep eating or stop. This training energizes careful part control and assists people with fostering a more prominent consciousness of their body's signs of yearning and completion.

The "slow-movement feast" is a careful eating exercise that welcomes people to eat a whole dinner in sluggish movement.

This conscious and purposeful methodology permits people to enjoy each nibble, notice the vibes of biting and gulping, and completely draw in with the eating system. This exercise supports an increased consciousness of the tactile experience of eating and advances a more careful and charming supper time.

The idea of "careful tastes" includes carrying care to the demonstration of drinking. Whether it's a warm cup of tea, a reviving glass of water, or any refreshment, people can rehearse careful tasting by focusing on the temperature, flavor, and sensations related with each taste. This exercise expands the standards of careful eating to refreshments, empowering people to relish and value the sustenance they give.

Careful strolling can be coordinated into the careful eating venture. This exercise includes going for a careful stroll previously or after a dinner, focusing on each step and the vibes of strolling. It fills in as an establishing practice that changes people into or out of the eating experience, encouraging a careful association between active work and sustenance.

The "five detects" practice urges people to connect each of the five faculties during feasts. Prior to taking a chomp, people can pause for a minute to see the varieties and show of the food (sight), appreciate the fragrance (smell), feel the surface of the food with their fingers (contact), pay attention to the sounds related with eating (hearing), and enjoy the flavors (taste). This far reaching exercise improves the tangible experience of eating and advances a more careful and purposeful way to deal with dinners.

Careful reflection is a significant activity that includes taking a couple of seconds after a dinner to consider the experience. People can think about the flavors, surfaces, and in general fulfillment of the feast. Furthermore, they can consider their degree of completion, any feelings or contemplations that emerged during dinner, and the decisions as far as part sizes and food determinations. This exercise supports mindfulness and can illuminate future careful eating rehearses.

The idea of "careful extravagance" includes permitting oneself to appreciate liberal or treat food varieties with care and without culpability. Rather than carelessly devouring these food sources, people can relish each chomp, focus on the sensations, and completely value the experience. This exercise advances a reasonable and non-prohibitive way to deal with eating, stressing care over judgment.

Careful shopping for food is an activity that stretches out the standards of care to the determination of fixings. Prior to putting things in the truck, people can pause for a minute to think about the dietary benefit, assortment, and generally speaking nature of the food sources they are picking. This exercise cultivates deliberateness in food choice and adds to a more careful and sustaining eating experience.

A careful eating exercise zeroed in on profound mindfulness includes focusing on close to home triggers that might impact dietary patterns. People can keep a careful eating diary, taking note of the feelings, contemplations, or circumstances that go before and go with dinners. This training energizes self-reflection and more prominent familiarity with the profound parts of eating, preparing for additional cognizant and purposeful decisions.

Careful cooking is an activity that includes carrying care to the course of feast planning. People can take part in deliberate activities, for example, cleaving vegetables, estimating fixings, and valuing the varieties and smells of the food. This training stretches out care to the whole food experience, from choice to arrangement, supporting the association between the cook and the sustenance gave.

The "careful respite" is an activity that urges people to take a short delay prior to going after seconds during a dinner. This delay permits people to check in with their body, survey their degree of completion, and settle on a cognizant conclusion about whether to eat. This training upholds careful part control and forestalls indulging by making space for mindfulness.

A careful eating exercise zeroed in on friendly associations includes rehearsing care during shared feasts. This exercise urges people to be completely present and participated in discussions, enjoying each nibble and valuing the organization of others. Careful eating in a social setting encourages a feeling of association and shared presence, adding to a more pleasant and careful feasting experience.

Careful eating rehearses are not inflexible standards but rather adaptable instruments that can be adjusted to individual inclinations and ways of life. As people investigate these activities, they might find which ones resound most with them and coordinate them into their everyday daily schedule. The key is to move toward careful eating with interest, transparency, and an eagerness to develop a more cognizant and purposeful relationship with food.

Careful eating activities and practices are necessary parts of a comprehensive way to deal with sustenance that goes past the simple demonstration of devouring food.

Established in the standards of care, these activities expect to develop an uplifted consciousness of the current second, advance deliberate decisions, and encourage a more profound association with the tangible experience of eating. Embracing these practices can add to a more offset and agreeable relationship with food, eventually improving by and large prosperity.

One fundamental careful eating exercise includes the act of careful breathing before dinners. This exercise fills in as an establishing procedure, empowering people to progress from the rushed speed of day to day existence to the current snapshot of eating. By taking a couple of purposeful breaths before the main nibble, people make a psychological shift, encouraging a feeling of quiet and presence. This deliberate breathing makes way for a more careful and purposeful way to deal with the dinner.

One more remarkable careful eating exercise is the act of eating without interruptions. In the period of steady availability and performing multiple tasks, numerous people have fostered the propensity for eating while at the same time sitting in front of the TV, looking at their telephones, or participating in different exercises. The activity of eating without interruptions welcomes people to make a devoted eating space liberated from electronic gadgets, permitting them to submerge themselves in the demonstration of eating completely. Eliminating outside interruptions supports an increased consciousness of the flavors, surfaces, and by and large tactile experience of the food, encouraging a more careful relationship with feasts.

Biting carefully is a clear yet effective activity that advances mindfulness during feasts. As opposed to hurrying through chomps, people are urged to zero in on the demonstration of biting, focusing on the surfaces and kinds of the food. This purposeful methodology upgrades the happiness regarding the dinner as well as supports better processing. Careful biting permits people to enjoy each nibble, making a seriously fulfilling and careful eating experience.

The raisin work out, an exemplary care practice, can be adjusted to careful eating. In this activity, people take a couple of seconds to notice a raisin prior to eating it intently. They note the variety, surface, and state of the raisin, connecting with their faculties completely. The training go on as they eat the raisin gradually, enjoying each nibble. This exercise supports an elevated consciousness of the tangible parts of eating and can be applied to different food varieties, cultivating a more profound association with the feeding demonstration of devouring food.

Rehearsing appreciation before feasts is a careful eating exercise that includes communicating appreciation for the food being devoured. Pausing for a minute to consider the excursion of the food from its source to the plate permits people to recognize the endeavors of those engaged with its creation. This exercise cultivates a feeling of appreciation for the sustenance the food gives and sets a good and careful tone prior to eating.

Careful part control is a strategy that urges people to be aware of serving sizes and focus on inside yearning and completion signals. The "plate stop" is an activity lined up with this idea. It includes having some time off partially through the feast to survey one's degree of completion. By putting down utensils, people can check in with their bodies, choosing whether to keep eating or stop. This training advances careful part control and assists people with fostering a more prominent consciousness of their body's signs, adding to better processing and generally prosperity.

The "slow-movement dinner" is a careful eating exercise that welcomes people to eat a whole feast in sluggish movement. This deliberate methodology permits people to appreciate each chomp, notice the impressions of biting and gulping, and completely draw in with the demonstration of eating.

The sluggish movement feast practice energizes an increased consciousness of the tangible experience of eating, advancing a more careful and charming supper time.

Careful tasting is a training that carries care to the demonstration of drinking. Whether it's a warm cup of tea, a reviving glass of water, or any drink, people can rehearse careful tasting by focusing on the temperature, flavor, and sensations related with each taste. This exercise broadens the standards of careful eating to drinks, empowering people to enjoy and value the sustenance gave.

Careful strolling can be consistently coordinated into the careful eating venture. This exercise includes going for a careful stroll previously or after a feast, focusing on each step and the impressions of strolling. It fills in as an establishing practice that changes people into or out of the eating experience, cultivating a careful association between actual work and sustenance.

The "five detects" practice urges people to connect every one of the five faculties during dinners. Prior to taking a chomp, people can pause for a minute to see the varieties and show of the food (sight), appreciate the fragrance (smell), feel the surface of the food with their fingers (contact), pay attention to the sounds related with eating (hearing), and relish the flavors (taste). This thorough activity improves the tactile experience of eating, advancing a more careful and deliberate way to deal with dinners.

Careful reflection is a significant activity that includes taking a couple of seconds after a feast to consider the experience. People can think about the flavors, surfaces, and by and large fulfillment of the feast. Also, they can think about their degree of completion, any feelings or contemplations that emerged during dinner, and the decisions as far as part sizes and food determinations. This exercise supports mindfulness and can illuminate future careful eating rehearses.

Careful extravagance is an activity that includes permitting oneself to appreciate liberal or treat food varieties with care and without culpability. Rather than carelessly eating these food varieties, people can relish each chomp, focus on the sensations, and completely value the experience. This exercise advances a reasonable and non-prohibitive way to deal with eating, underlining care over judgment.

Careful shopping for food is an activity that stretches out the standards of care to the determination of fixings. Prior to putting things in the truck, people can pause for a minute to think about the dietary benefit, assortment, and generally nature of the food sources they are picking. This exercise cultivates deliberateness in food choice and adds to a more careful and supporting eating experience.

Embracing a careful cooking practice includes carrying care to the course of dinner readiness. People can take part in purposeful activities, for example, cleaving vegetables, estimating fixings, and valuing the varieties and smells of the food. This training stretches out care to the whole food experience, from determination to planning, building up the association between the cook and the sustenance gave.

The "careful interruption" is an activity that urges people to take a short delay prior to going after seconds during a feast. This purposeful delay permits people to check in with their bodies, survey their degree of completion, and settle on a cognizant conclusion about whether to eat. This training upholds careful part control and forestalls indulging by making space for mindfulness.

A careful eating exercise zeroed in on close to home mindfulness includes focusing on profound triggers that might impact dietary patterns. People can keep a careful eating diary, noticing the feelings, considerations, or circumstances that go before and go with feasts. This training energizes self-reflection and a more prominent familiarity with the profound parts of eating, preparing for additional cognizant and deliberate decisions.

Careful eating in a social setting is an activity that includes rehearsing care during shared feasts. This exercise urges people to be completely present and participated in discussions, relishing each nibble and valuing the organization of others. Careful eating in a group environment encourages a feeling of association and shared presence, adding to a more pleasant and careful feasting experience.

As people investigate these careful eating works out, they might find which ones resound most with them and incorporate them into their day to day daily schedule. It is significant to move toward careful eating with interest, transparency, and a readiness to develop a more cognizant and deliberate relationship with food. These activities are not inflexible principles but rather adaptable apparatuses that can be adjusted to individual inclinations and ways of life.

All in all, careful eating activities and practices offer a different exhibit of devices for people trying to upgrade their mindfulness during dinners. These activities, well established in the standards of care, energize purposeful decisions, tactile commitment, and a significant association with the supporting demonstration of devouring food. Whether through careful breathing, purposeful biting, or intelligent practices, these activities add to a more offset and agreeable relationship with food, cultivating in general prosperity and a careful way to deal with sustenance.

Chapter 7

Personalized Nutrition

Customized nourishment is a quickly developing field that tailors dietary proposals to individual qualities like hereditary qualities, way of life, and wellbeing status. The idea comes from the acknowledgment that one-size-fits-all dietary exhortation may not be successful for everybody, given the innate changeability in human science and digestion. This approach stands out from conventional dietary rules, which frequently give general proposals appropriate to the whole populace.

At the center of customized nourishment is the possibility that people answer diversely to similar food varieties in view of their special hereditary cosmetics. Progresses in genomic research have divulged a heap of hereditary varieties that impact how our bodies cycle and use supplements. These varieties, known as single nucleotide polymorphisms (SNPs), can affect catalysts, receptors, and other sub-atomic parts engaged with digestion. By understanding these hereditary subtleties, specialists expect to tailor dietary plans that improve supplement ingestion and usage for every individual.

Notwithstanding hereditary qualities, customized nourishment considers different way of life factors, including active work, rest designs, feelings of anxiety, and dietary inclinations. These variables add to the perplexing transaction of components impacting a person's wholesome requirements. For example, somebody with a stationary way of life might require an unexpected supplement profile in comparison to a competitor participated in thorough preparation. Also, people with high-feelings of anxiety might profit from dietary suggestions that help mental prosperity.

Progressions in innovation, especially in the fields of genomics and information examination, have worked with the rise of customized sustenance. Hereditary testing, for instance, has become more open and reasonable, permitting people to get experiences into their hereditary inclinations connected with nourishment. Investigating this hereditary data close by other way of life information empowers the production of customized nourishment plans.

Nutrigenomics, a part of wholesome genomics, researches what qualities mean for a singular's reaction to supplements and what supplements mean for quality articulation. This interdisciplinary field consolidates hereditary qualities, nourishment, and sub-atomic science to disentangle the multifaceted associations among hereditary qualities and dietary examples. Nutrigenomics plans to recognize explicit dietary proposals in view of a person's hereditary cosmetics to advance ideal wellbeing and forestall or oversee different circumstances.

The use of customized sustenance reaches out past wellbeing advancement and sickness avoidance; it is progressively being investigated in the administration of persistent illnesses. Conditions like diabetes, cardiovascular sicknesses, and heftiness display critical heterogeneity among people. Customized sustenance methodologies expect to address this heterogeneity by fitting dietary mediations to the particular requirements of every patient, possibly further developing treatment results and long haul wellbeing.

With regards to weight the board, customized sustenance thinks about elements like digestion, satiety reactions, and the stomach microbiome. The stomach microbiome, a complicated environment of microorganisms living in the gastrointestinal system, assumes a significant part in supplement digestion and generally wellbeing. Research proposes that the organization of the stomach microbiome can impact how people answer different dietary examples. Customized sustenance procedures might include balancing the stomach microbiota through designated dietary intercessions to help weight the executives objectives.

Besides, arising research demonstrates that the planning of food consumption, known as chrono-sustenance, may likewise assume a part in customized nourishment. The body's circadian musicality, the interior organic clock managing different physiological cycles more than a 24-hour cycle, impacts supplement digestion and energy consumption. Customized nourishment plans might consider the person's circadian cadence to advance the planning of dinners and upgrade metabolic wellbeing.

Regardless of the promising capability of customized nourishment, challenges and moral contemplations go with its execution. Security concerns connected with hereditary information, the precision of hereditary testing, and the potential for belittling in light of hereditary inclinations are significant perspectives to address. Additionally, the interpretation of logical discoveries into significant and useful dietary suggestions requires progressing exploration and approval.

The incorporation of customized nourishment into standard medical services likewise brings up issues about availability and moderateness. While hereditary testing has become more open, differences in admittance to medical services assets might restrict the far and wide reception of customized sustenance draws near. Connecting these holes is fundamental to guarantee that the advantages of customized sustenance are accessible to assorted populaces.

In the domain of general wellbeing, customized nourishment can possibly upset sustenance arrangements and mediations. Creating some distance from nonexclusive dietary rules could prompt more designated and compelling methodologies for forestalling diet-related illnesses. States and wellbeing associations might have to adjust their ways to deal with sustenance training and general wellbeing efforts to integrate customized nourishment standards.

Teaching medical services experts about customized nourishment is one more basic part of its reconciliation into medical services frameworks. Doctors, dietitians, and other medical services suppliers should be furnished with the information and devices to decipher and apply customized nourishment data in clinical settings. Proficient improvement programs and instructive assets can assume a critical part in getting ready medical services experts for the time of customized medication.

The job of man-made reasoning (artificial intelligence) and AI in customized nourishment is an area of dynamic investigation. These advancements can break down huge datasets, including hereditary data, way of life variables, and wellbeing records, to distinguish designs and produce customized suggestions. Man-made intelligence calculations can persistently learn and adjust in light of individual reactions, refining proposals over the long haul. While the potential advantages are significant, moral contemplations encompassing information security, calculation straightforwardness, and informed assent should be painstakingly tended to.

In the customer domain, the prominence of customized sustenance is obvious in the ascent of direct-to-buyer hereditary testing administrations and customized dinner arranging applications. These devices engage people to assume command over their wellbeing by giving customized bits of knowledge and proposals. Be that as it may, the precision and dependability of these administrations differ, and shoppers ought to move toward them with a basic eye. Moreover, the translation of hereditary data might require direction from medical services experts to guarantee informed navigation.

Social and dietary variety add one more layer of intricacy to the execution of customized sustenance on a worldwide scale. Various populaces have unmistakable dietary propensities, inclinations, and hereditary varieties. Tweaking sustenance suggestions to suit assorted social settings is critical to guarantee the pertinence and viability of customized nourishment systems around the world.

As customized sustenance keeps on developing, interdisciplinary cooperation among researchers, medical services experts, policymakers, and innovation specialists is central. The joining of mastery from different fields is vital for address the multilayered parts of customized sustenance, from genomics and microbial science to morals and general wellbeing.

All in all, customized sustenance addresses a change in perspective by they way we approach dietary suggestions and wellbeing mediations. By recognizing and embracing individual inconstancy, customized nourishment can possibly upgrade wellbeing results, forestall persistent illnesses, and reform the eventual fate of sustenance and medical services. As exploration and innovation keep on propelling, the vision of a customized way to deal with nourishment might turn into a basic part of advancing wellbeing and prosperity on a worldwide scale.

7.1 Exploring the idea that there is no one-size-fits-all approach to nutrition.

The idea of a one-size-fits-all way to deal with nourishment has for quite some time been implanted in customary dietary rules and general wellbeing proposals. In any case, a developing group of proof and a change in logical reasoning are testing this idea, proposing that singular fluctuation in hereditary qualities, digestion, and way of life requires a more customized way to deal with sustenance. This investigation dives into the possibility that there is no widespread remedy for ideal sustenance and considers the variables adding to the individualized idea of dietary necessities.

At the core of the contention against a one-size-fits-all approach is the acknowledgment of human hereditary variety. Hereditary varieties among people can essentially influence how the body processes and uses supplements. The field of nutrigenomics investigates this multifaceted interchange among hereditary qualities and sustenance, intending to recognize how explicit hereditary variables impact a singular's reaction to various food varieties.

Single nucleotide polymorphisms (SNPs), varieties in a solitary DNA building block, are among the hereditary elements explored in nutrigenomics. These varieties can influence proteins, receptors, and other sub-atomic parts associated with supplement digestion. For example, an individual might have a hereditary inclination that impacts their capacity to effectively use specific nutrients or minerals. By understanding these hereditary subtleties, customized nourishment tries to fit dietary proposals to address individual necessities and enhance supplement use.

Past hereditary qualities, way of life factors contribute essentially to the fluctuation in wholesome necessities. Active work levels, occupation, rest designs, feelings of anxiety, and dietary inclinations all assume a part in molding a person's wholesome necessities. For instance, a competitor participated in serious preparation might require an alternate supplement profile contrasted with a stationary person. Essentially, somebody with a high-stress occupation might profit from dietary suggestions that help pressure the executives and mental prosperity.

Progressions in innovation, especially in the fields of genomics and information examination, have made ready for customized nourishment. Hereditary testing, when an expensive and complex method, has become more open and reasonable. People can now get experiences into their hereditary inclinations connected with sustenance, considering a more educated and fitted way to deal with dietary decisions. Examining this hereditary data close by information on way of life factors empowers the production of customized nourishment designs that think about both hereditary and natural impacts.

The field of nutrigenomics, with its emphasis on understanding how qualities connect with supplements, has given important bits of knowledge into customized nourishment. Specialists intend to distinguish explicit hereditary markers related with reactions to dietary parts like starches, fats, and nutrients. This information can then be utilized to foster designated dietary suggestions in light of a person's hereditary cosmetics, fully intent on advancing ideal wellbeing and forestalling diet-related illnesses.

With regards to persistent illnesses, customized sustenance holds critical commitment. Conditions like diabetes, cardiovascular illnesses, and heftiness show extensive heterogeneity among people. Customary treatment approaches frequently depend on summed up dietary suggestions, however customized nourishment methodologies mean to address this heterogeneity by fitting mediations to the particular requirements of every patient. This individualized methodology might prompt more compelling illness the executives and further developed wellbeing results.

Weight the executives is another region where customized nourishment can have a significant effect. Factors like digestion, satiety reactions, and the stomach microbiome add to the mind boggling nature of weight guideline. Research recommends that the sythesis of the stomach microbiome, the local area of microorganisms in the gastrointestinal system, can impact how people answer different dietary examples. Customized sustenance procedures might include regulating the stomach microbiota through designated dietary intercessions to help weight the board objectives.

The idea of chrono-sustenance, taking into account the planning of food consumption, is getting momentum inside the domain of customized nourishment. The body's circadian mood, the inside natural clock that manages different physiological cycles more than a 24-hour cycle, impacts supplement digestion and energy consumption. Customized sustenance plans might consider a person's circadian beat to upgrade the planning of dinners, possibly improving metabolic wellbeing.

Notwithstanding the promising capability of customized sustenance, a few difficulties and moral contemplations should be tended to. Protection concerns connected with hereditary information, the precision of hereditary testing, and the potential for trashing in view of hereditary inclinations are basic angles to consider. In addition, making an interpretation of logical discoveries into noteworthy and reasonable dietary suggestions requires continuous exploration and approval.

The mix of customized sustenance into standard medical care brings up issues about openness and reasonableness. While hereditary testing has become more open, there are variations in admittance to medical care assets that might restrict the boundless reception of customized nourishment draws near. Guaranteeing that the advantages of customized sustenance are accessible to assorted populaces is fundamental for address wellbeing imbalances.

In the domain of general wellbeing, customized sustenance can possibly reform nourishment strategies and mediations. Getting away from nonexclusive dietary rules could prompt more designated and powerful methodologies for forestalling diet-related sicknesses. Legislatures and wellbeing associations might have to adjust their ways to deal with sustenance instruction and general wellbeing efforts to consolidate customized nourishment standards.

Instructing medical care experts about customized nourishment is one more basic part of its reconciliation into medical services frameworks. Doctors, dietitians, and other medical services suppliers should be furnished with the information and devices to decipher and apply customized nourishment data in clinical settings. Proficient improvement programs and instructive assets can assume a vital part in getting ready medical care experts for the time of customized medication.

The job of computerized reasoning (artificial intelligence) and AI in customized sustenance is an area of dynamic investigation. These advancements can break down tremendous datasets, including hereditary data, way of life elements, and wellbeing records, to distinguish designs and produce customized proposals. Artificial intelligence calculations can constantly learn and adjust in view of individual reactions, refining suggestions over the long run. While the potential advantages are significant, moral contemplations encompassing information security, calculation straightforwardness, and informed assent should be painstakingly tended to.

In the buyer domain, the prevalence of customized sustenance is clear in the ascent of direct-to-purchaser hereditary testing administrations and customized dinner arranging applications. These instruments engage people to assume command over their wellbeing by giving customized bits of knowledge and suggestions. In any case, the exactness and dependability of these administrations shift, and customers ought to move toward them with a basic eye. Also, the translation of hereditary data might require direction from medical care experts to guarantee informed navigation.

Social and dietary variety add one more layer of intricacy to the execution of customized sustenance on a worldwide scale. Various populaces have unmistakable dietary propensities, inclinations, and hereditary varieties. Tweaking sustenance proposals to suit different social settings is vital to guarantee the pertinence and adequacy of customized nourishment systems around the world.

As customized nourishment keeps on advancing, interdisciplinary cooperation among researchers, medical care experts, policymakers, and innovation specialists is vital. The incorporation of aptitude from different fields is fundamental for address the multi-layered parts of customized nourishment, from genomics and microbial science to morals and general wellbeing.

All in all, the investigation of the possibility that there is nobody size-fits-all way to deal with sustenance uncovers a change in outlook by they way we see and move toward dietary suggestions. Recognizing and embracing individual fluctuation, customized sustenance can possibly advance wellbeing results, forestall constant sicknesses, and rethink the eventual fate of nourishment and medical services. As exploration and innovation keep on propelling, the vision of a customized way to deal with sustenance might turn into a major part of advancing wellbeing and prosperity on a worldwide scale.

7.2 Discussing genetic factors, individual differences.

Understanding the job of hereditary variables and individual contrasts in different parts of human existence has been a focal point of logical request for a really long time. With regards to wellbeing and sustenance, this investigation turns out to be especially pivotal. This conversation dives into the perplexing transaction between hereditary qualities, individual contrasts, and their effect on wellbeing, with a particular accentuation on how these variables impact reactions to count calories and dietary intercessions.

Hereditary variables assume a basic part in molding a singular's inclination to different medical issue and their reactions to outside upgrades, including dietary examples. The Human Genome Undertaking, finished in 2003, denoted a critical achievement in hereditary exploration by planning the whole human genome. This fantastic accomplishment made ready for a more profound comprehension of the hereditary premise of wellbeing and illness, establishing the groundwork for resulting research in nutrigenomics — the investigation of what individual hereditary varieties mean for reactions to supplements.

Single nucleotide polymorphisms (SNPs) are one of the key hereditary elements researched in nutrigenomics. SNPs address varieties in a solitary DNA building block, and they can impact how the body processes and uses supplements. These hereditary varieties might influence proteins, receptors, and other sub-atomic parts engaged with digestion, in this way forming a person's healthful necessities.

For example, a few people might convey hereditary varieties that influence their capacity to productively process specific nutrients or minerals. The MTHFR quality, engaged with the digestion of folate, is a very much concentrated on model. Certain variations of the MTHFR quality might affect folate digestion, possibly impacting defenselessness to conditions, for example, brain tube surrenders and cardiovascular infection. Seeing such hereditary subtleties considers a more customized way to deal with sustenance, fitting dietary proposals to address individual hereditary inclinations.

The field of nutrigenomics means to recognize explicit hereditary markers related with reactions to various dietary parts.

Research centers around understanding how qualities cooperate with macronutrients (sugars, fats, proteins) and micronutrients (nutrients, minerals) to impact wellbeing results. By interpreting these hereditary cooperations, researchers endeavor to foster designated dietary proposals in view of a person's hereditary cosmetics.

Individual contrasts stretch out past hereditary qualities to incorporate many elements, including way of life, climate, and individual decisions. Way of life factors, for example, active work, rest designs, feelings of anxiety, and dietary inclinations contribute essentially to the complicated transaction of components molding a person's wholesome requirements. These variables communicate with hereditary inclinations, making an extraordinary profile that impacts how the body answers dietary mediations.

Actual work, for instance, has significant ramifications for nourishing prerequisites. Competitors participated in thorough preparation might have expanded energy and supplement requests contrasted with stationary people. The sort and power of actual work can affect supplement digestion, impacting the requirement for explicit supplements like carbs, proteins, and micronutrients. Individualizing dietary proposals in view of action levels is vital for help ideal execution and recuperation.

Rest designs likewise assume an essential part in by and large wellbeing and digestion. Disturbances in rest can influence hunger directing chemicals, prompting changes in food desires and energy balance. People with unpredictable rest examples might encounter modifications in glucose digestion and insulin awareness, impacting their reaction to various dietary examples. Taking into account individual rest propensities becomes significant while fitting sustenance intends to advance by and large prosperity.

Stress, both intense and ongoing, addresses another singular contrast that can influence dietary necessities. The body's reaction to push includes the arrival of chemicals, for example, cortisol, which can impact hunger, food decisions, and digestion. Persistent pressure might add to gorging or picking energy-thick, supplement unfortunate food sources, possibly influencing weight the executives and generally speaking wellbeing. Tending to pressure as a component of customized sustenance procedures is fundamental for exhaustive prosperity.

Dietary inclinations and social impacts add to the variety of individual nourishing necessities. Various populaces have unmistakable dietary propensities and inclinations in view of social customs, food accessibility, and financial variables. Customized nourishment considers these social varieties, perceiving that dietary suggestions should line up with people's inclinations and ways of life to be feasible and successful.

Progressions in innovation play had an essential impact in opening the capability of customized nourishment.

Hereditary testing, when a complicated and costly methodology, has become more open, permitting people to get experiences into their hereditary inclinations connected with sustenance. Direct-to-customer hereditary testing administrations offer the accommodation of investigating one's hereditary cosmetics and getting customized experiences into different wellbeing angles, including nourishment.

Dissecting hereditary data close by other way of life information empowers the production of customized nourishment plans. These plans think about both hereditary and ecological variables, giving an all encompassing way to deal with upgrading nourishing results. The reconciliation of innovation and information investigation works with the union of immense measures of data, considering the recognizable proof of examples and patterns that illuminate customized dietary proposals.

The stomach microbiome, a perplexing biological system of microorganisms living in the intestinal system, addresses one more element of individual fluctuation in sustenance. The organization of the stomach microbiome changes among people, impacted by variables like hereditary qualities, diet, and climate. Research recommends that the stomach microbiome assumes an essential part in supplement digestion, resistant capability, and generally wellbeing.

The stomach microbiome impacts how the body ingests, processes, and uses supplements from the eating routine. It additionally adds to the creation of specific nutrients and bioactive mixtures. Customized sustenance systems might include considering the singular's stomach microbiome profile while fitting dietary proposals. Adjusting the stomach microbiota through designated dietary intercessions, like the utilization of probiotics or prebiotics, is an area of dynamic exploration with the possibility to advance wellbeing results.

With regards to ongoing sicknesses, individual contrasts in hereditary vulnerability and way of life factors add to the heterogeneity saw in illness appearance and movement. For instance, people with a family background of diabetes might have a higher hereditary inclination to the condition. Customized nourishment techniques for diabetes the board would then think about both hereditary variables and way of life components like dietary propensities, active work, and weight the executives.

Cardiovascular infections likewise display critical fluctuation among people. Hereditary variables might impact cholesterol digestion, circulatory strain guideline, and other cardiovascular gamble factors. Fitting dietary proposals to address these hereditary inclinations, joined with way of life changes, can assume a urgent part in forestalling and overseeing cardiovascular sicknesses on an individualized premise.

Heftiness, a perplexing condition impacted by hereditary, natural, and conduct factors, highlights the significance of customized sustenance in weight the executives.

Hereditary varieties can affect digestion, craving guideline, and fat stockpiling, adding to individual contrasts in powerlessness to weight. Customized nourishment systems might include tending to these hereditary elements close by conduct and way of life intercessions to help practical weight reduction.

Weight the executives isn't just about caloric equilibrium yet in addition about understanding how a singular's body answers different dietary examples. A few people might encounter improved results with low-carb eats less, while others might answer all the more well to low-fat weight control plans. Customized nourishment recognizes these singular distinctions and designers dietary suggestions to upgrade weight the executives in light of hereditary, metabolic, and way of life factors.

The arising field of chrono-nourishment further features the significance of individual contrasts in the planning of food consumption. The body's circadian musicality, the inward organic clock that directs different physiological cycles more than a 24-hour cycle, impacts supplement digestion and energy use. Customized nourishment plans might consider a person's circadian musicality to upgrade the planning of dinners, possibly improving metabolic wellbeing and weight guideline.

Regardless of the promising capability of customized sustenance, challenges and moral contemplations go with its execution. Protection concerns connected with hereditary information, the exactness of hereditary testing, and the potential for derision in light of hereditary inclinations are significant viewpoints to address. Additionally, making an interpretation of logical discoveries into significant and useful dietary proposals requires continuous exploration and approval.

The mix of customized nourishment into standard medical care brings up issues about openness and moderateness. While hereditary testing has become more open, there are differences in admittance to medical care assets that might restrict the broad reception of customized sustenance draws near. Guaranteeing that the advantages of customized nourishment are accessible to different populaces is crucial for address wellbeing disparities.

In the domain of general wellbeing, customized nourishment can possibly upset sustenance strategies and mediations. Creating some distance from nonexclusive dietary rules could prompt more designated and compelling procedures for forestalling diet-related illnesses. States and wellbeing associations might have to adjust their ways to deal with nourishment instruction and general wellbeing efforts to integrate customized sustenance standards.

Teaching medical care experts about customized nourishment is one more basic part of its mix into medical care frameworks.

Doctors, dietitians, and other medical care suppliers should be furnished with the information and apparatuses to decipher and apply customized nourishment data in clinical settings. Proficient improvement programs and instructive assets can assume a crucial part in planning medical care experts for the time of customized medication.

The job of man-made brainpower (man-made intelligence) and AI in customized sustenance is an area of dynamic investigation. These innovations can examine tremendous datasets, including hereditary data, way of life variables, and wellbeing records, to distinguish designs and produce customized suggestions. Simulated intelligence calculations can persistently learn and adjust in view of individual reactions, refining proposals after some time. While the potential advantages are significant, moral contemplations encompassing information security, calculation straightforwardness, and informed assent should be painstakingly tended to.

In the purchaser domain, the prominence of customized sustenance is obvious in the ascent of direct-to-shopper hereditary testing administrations and customized feast arranging applications. These devices enable people to assume command over their wellbeing by giving customized bits of knowledge and proposals. Notwithstanding, the precision and dependability of these administrations differ, and shoppers ought to move toward them with a basic eye. Furthermore, the translation of hereditary data might require direction from medical care experts to guarantee informed navigation.

Social and dietary variety add one more layer of intricacy to the execution of customized nourishment on a worldwide scale. Various populaces have particular dietary propensities, inclinations, and hereditary varieties. Altering sustenance proposals to suit different social settings is essential to guarantee the pertinence and adequacy of customized nourishment techniques around the world.

As customized nourishment keeps on developing, interdisciplinary joint effort among researchers, medical care experts, policymakers, and innovation specialists is central. The mix of mastery from different fields is crucial for address the diverse parts of customized sustenance, from genomics and microbial science to morals and general wellbeing.

All in all, the conversation on hereditary variables and individual contrasts in sustenance highlights the requirement for a change in outlook by they way we approach dietary suggestions and wellbeing mediations. Perceiving and embracing the intricacy of individual inconstancy, customized sustenance can possibly upgrade wellbeing results, forestall constant illnesses, and rethink the eventual fate of nourishment and medical services. As examination and innovation keep on propelling, the vision of a customized way to deal with sustenance might turn into an essential part of advancing wellbeing and prosperity on a worldwide scale.

7.3 The importance of adapting dietary choices to personal needs and preferences.

Dietary decisions assume a crucial part in molding our general wellbeing and prosperity. The food sources we eat give fundamental supplements that fuel our bodies, support development, and keep up with different physiological capabilities. Customarily, dietary suggestions have frequently followed a one-size-fits-all methodology, expecting that a uniform arrangement of rules is reasonable for everybody. In any case, a rising collection of proof recommends that customized nourishment, which adjusts dietary decisions to individual requirements and inclinations, might be a more viable and economical methodology for advancing wellbeing.

One of the essential parts of adjusting dietary decisions to individual requirements is perceiving the variety among people. Every individual has a novel hereditary cosmetics, way of life, and wellbeing status that add to varieties in nourishing prerequisites. Hereditary elements, specifically, can impact how our bodies utilize and answer various supplements. The arising field of nutrigenomics investigates these hereditary varieties to tailor dietary proposals in light of a person's hereditary profile.

Understanding hereditary variables takes into consideration a more exact and designated way to deal with nourishment. For instance, people might have hereditary varieties that influence their capacity to proficiently utilize specific supplements. The consideration of hereditary data in customized sustenance methodologies empowers the distinguishing proof of explicit dietary examples that line up with a person's hereditary inclinations, advancing supplement retention and use.

Way of life factors likewise assume a critical part in deciding a person's nourishing necessities. Factors, for example, actual work, rest designs, feelings of anxiety, and occupation add to the perplexing transaction of components that impact dietary necessities. Fitting dietary decisions to oblige these way of life factors guarantees that nourishing proposals line up with a singular's day to day exercises, energy use, and generally prosperity.

Active work, specifically, is a critical determinant of dietary requirements. Competitors participated in thorough preparation have higher energy and supplement prerequisites contrasted with stationary people. Customized sustenance for competitors thinks about elements like the kind of movement, power, and length, giving a designated way to deal with filling execution, advancing recuperation, and forestalling supplement lacks.

Rest designs likewise influence dietary decisions and healthful digestion. Disturbances in rest can impact hunger directing chemicals, possibly prompting changes in food inclinations and energy balance. People with sporadic rest examples might encounter adjustments in glucose digestion and insulin awareness, featuring the significance of integrating rest contemplations into customized nourishment plans.

Stress, whether intense or ongoing, addresses another way of life factor impacting dietary decisions. The body's reaction to stretch includes the arrival of chemicals that can affect hunger, food decisions, and digestion. People encountering elevated degrees of stress might be inclined to gorging or choosing solace food sources, affecting their generally speaking wholesome admission. Customized nourishment considers feelings of anxiety, offering techniques to help pressure the board through dietary decisions.

Besides, dietary inclinations and social impacts contribute essentially to the variety of individual healthful necessities. Customized sustenance perceives that one's social foundation, food inclinations, and dietary propensities are indispensable to making practical and pleasant dietary plans. Adjusting healthful suggestions to individual preferences and social practices upgrades adherence to dietary plans, making them more plausible in the long haul.

Headways in innovation, especially in the field of hereditary testing and information examination, have made ready for the combination of customized nourishment into standard wellbeing rehearses. Hereditary testing, when a complicated and exorbitant strategy, has become more open, permitting people to acquire experiences into their hereditary inclinations connected with sustenance. Dissecting hereditary data close by way of life information empowers the formation of customized nourishment designs that think about both hereditary and ecological impacts.

The stomach microbiome, a unique local area of microorganisms living in the gastrointestinal system, adds one more layer to the intricacy of customizing sustenance. The structure of the stomach microbiome differs among people and can be impacted by hereditary qualities, diet, and ecological elements. Research recommends that the stomach microbiome assumes a pivotal part in supplement digestion, safe capability, and generally wellbeing.

Customized nourishment methodologies might include considering a singular's stomach microbiome profile while fitting dietary proposals. Tweaking the stomach microbiota through designated dietary mediations, like the incorporation of probiotics or prebiotics, can be essential for a customized way to deal with help stomach well-being and streamline supplement retention.

With regards to persistent illnesses, adjusting dietary decisions to individual requirements is especially pertinent. Conditions like diabetes, cardiovascular illnesses, and heftiness display critical heterogeneity among people. Customized sustenance techniques expect to address this heterogeneity by fitting dietary intercessions to the particular necessities of every patient, possibly further developing treatment results and long haul wellbeing.

For people with diabetes, customized sustenance includes considering variables, for example, insulin awareness, blood glucose levels, and individual reactions to various carbs. Fitting carb admission to line up with a person's glycemic reaction assists in advancing with blooding sugar control.

Customized sustenance plans for cardiovascular wellbeing might zero in on dietary examples that address explicit gamble factors, for example, raised cholesterol levels or hypertension.

Weight the executives is one more region where adjusting dietary decisions to individual necessities is vital. Hereditary varieties can impact digestion, craving guideline, and reactions to various macronutrients. Customized nourishment recognizes these singular distinctions and designers dietary suggestions to help feasible weight reduction or upkeep. This might include changing macronutrient proportions, taking into account the planning of dinners, and tending to mental parts of eating conduct.

The idea of chrono-sustenance, which thinks about the planning of food consumption, further underlines the significance of adjusting dietary decisions to circadian rhythms. The body's circadian cadence impacts supplement digestion and energy use north of a 24-hour cycle. Customized nourishment plans might consider a person's circadian beat to advance the planning of dinners, possibly working on metabolic wellbeing and supporting weight guideline.

Notwithstanding the promising capability of customized nourishment, challenges and moral contemplations should be tended to. Protection concerns connected with hereditary information, the exactness of hereditary testing, and the potential for trashing in light of hereditary inclinations are significant angles to consider. Also, the interpretation of logical discoveries into significant and pragmatic dietary suggestions requires continuous examination and approval.

The reconciliation of customized sustenance into standard medical services brings up issues about availability and reasonableness. While hereditary testing has become more available, there are variations in admittance to medical care assets that might restrict the broad reception of customized nourishment draws near. Guaranteeing that the advantages of customized sustenance are accessible to assorted populaces is crucial for address wellbeing imbalances.

In the domain of general wellbeing, customized sustenance can possibly alter nourishment approaches and mediations. Getting away from conventional dietary rules could prompt more designated and successful methodologies for forestalling diet-related illnesses. Legislatures and wellbeing associations might have to adjust their ways to deal with sustenance training and general wellbeing efforts to integrate customized nourishment standards.

Instructing medical care experts about customized nourishment is one more basic part of its joining into medical care frameworks. Doctors, dietitians, and other medical care suppliers should be outfitted with the information and apparatuses to decipher and apply customized nourishment data in clinical settings. Proficient improvement programs and instructive assets can assume a significant part in getting ready medical care experts for the time of customized medication.

In the purchaser domain, the ubiquity of customized nourishment is apparent in the ascent of direct-to-shopper hereditary testing administrations and customized feast arranging applications. These instruments enable people to assume command over their wellbeing by giving customized bits of knowledge and proposals. In any case, the precision and dependability of these administrations change, and purchasers ought to move toward them with a basic eye. Also, the translation of hereditary data might require direction from medical services experts to guarantee informed navigation.

Social and dietary variety add one more layer of intricacy to the execution of customized sustenance on a worldwide scale. Various populaces have unmistakable dietary propensities, inclinations, and hereditary varieties. Tweaking nourishment proposals to suit different social settings is vital to guarantee the pertinence and adequacy of customized sustenance methodologies around the world.

The idea of adjusting dietary decisions to individual requirements and inclinations is a principal part of advancing comprehensive wellbeing and prosperity. In the domain of sustenance, perceiving and embracing individual variety is significant, recognizing that there is nobody size-fits-all way to deal with what comprises an ideal eating regimen. This conversation digs into the complex parts of individual requirements and inclinations with regards to nourishment, traversing hereditary variables, way of life contemplations, social impacts, and the arising field of customized sustenance.

Hereditary variables structure a foundation in the scene of customized nourishment. Every individual's hereditary cosmetics adds to their interesting digestion, supplement necessities, and reactions to different dietary parts. The field of nutrigenomics investigates the mind boggling connection among hereditary qualities and sustenance, intending to unwind how explicit hereditary varieties impact a singular's reaction to various food varieties.

Single nucleotide polymorphisms (SNPs) are key hereditary varieties explored in nutrigenomics. These varieties, happening in a solitary DNA building block, can influence proteins, receptors, and other sub-atomic parts engaged with supplement digestion. For example, varieties in qualities connected with carb digestion might impact how a singular cycles sugars and starches. By understanding these hereditary subtleties, customized nourishment tries to tailor dietary suggestions to upgrade supplement assimilation and usage for every individual.

The coordination of hereditary data into customized nourishment techniques considers a more exact comprehension of a person's dietary necessities. Hereditary testing, when an intricate and costly system, has become more open, empowering people to acquire bits of knowledge into their hereditary inclinations connected with sustenance. This data, joined with information on way of life factors, works with the making of customized nourishment designs that think about both hereditary and ecological impacts.

Way of life factors address one more element of individual necessities and inclinations in nourishment. Actual work, rest designs, feelings of anxiety, and occupation contribute altogether to the intricacy of dietary prerequisites. Perceiving and adjusting dietary decisions to oblige these way of life factors guarantees that healthful proposals line up with a singular's everyday exercises, energy use, and generally speaking prosperity.

Actual work, specifically, assumes a focal part in molding nourishing necessities. Competitors participated in concentrated preparing have raised energy and supplement necessities contrasted with stationary people. Customized sustenance for competitors thinks about elements like the kind of action, power, and span, giving a designated way to deal with energizing execution, supporting recuperation, and forestalling supplement inadequacies.

Rest designs additionally impact dietary decisions and nourishing digestion. Disturbances in rest can affect hunger controlling chemicals, possibly prompting changes in food inclinations and energy balance. People with unpredictable rest examples might encounter changes in glucose digestion and insulin awareness, highlighting the significance of integrating rest contemplations into customized sustenance plans.

Stress, whether intense or persistent, addresses another way of life factor impacting dietary decisions. The body's reaction to push includes the arrival of chemicals that can influence craving, food decisions, and digestion. People encountering elevated degrees of stress might be inclined to indulging or choosing solace food varieties, impacting their by and large healthful admission. Customized sustenance considers feelings of anxiety, offering systems to help pressure the executives through dietary decisions.

Dietary inclinations and social impacts contribute fundamentally to the variety of individual wholesome requirements. Customized sustenance perceives that one's social foundation, food inclinations, and dietary propensities are indispensable to making supportable and charming dietary plans. Adjusting wholesome proposals to individual preferences and social practices upgrades adherence to dietary plans, making them more doable in the long haul.

The interaction between hereditary qualities, way of life elements, and dietary inclinations highlights the intricacy of customizing sustenance. Headways in innovation, especially in hereditary testing and information examination, have worked with the coordination of these different elements into customized sustenance draws near. The stomach microbiome, a unique local area of microorganisms living in the gastro-intestinal system, adds one more layer to the intricacy of customizing sustenance.

The stomach microbiome fluctuates among people and can be impacted by hereditary qualities, diet, and ecological elements. Research proposes that the stomach microbiome assumes a pivotal part in supplement digestion, resistant capability, and by and large wellbeing.

Customized sustenance procedures might include considering a singular's stomach microbiome profile while fitting dietary proposals. Tweaking the stomach microbiota through designated dietary mediations, like the incorporation of probiotics or prebiotics, can be essential for a customized way to deal with help stomach wellbeing and improve supplement retention.

With regards to constant illnesses, adjusting dietary decisions to individual necessities is especially applicable. Conditions like diabetes, cardiovascular infections, and weight show huge heterogeneity among people. Customized nourishment methodologies plan to address this heterogeneity by fitting dietary intercessions to the particular requirements of every patient, possibly further developing treatment results and long haul wellbeing.

For people with diabetes, customized sustenance includes considering elements, for example, insulin awareness, blood glucose levels, and individual reactions to various sugars. Fitting starch admission to line up with a person's glycemic reaction assists in improving with blooding sugar control. Customized sustenance plans for cardiovascular wellbeing might zero in on dietary examples that address explicit gamble factors, for example, raised cholesterol levels or hypertension.

Weight the executives is one more region where adjusting dietary decisions to individual necessities is urgent. Hereditary varieties can impact digestion, craving guideline, and reactions to various macronutrients. Customized sustenance recognizes these singular distinctions and designers dietary proposals to help manageable weight reduction or support. This might include changing macronutrient proportions, taking into account the planning of feasts, and tending to mental parts of eating conduct.

The idea of chrono-sustenance, which thinks about the planning of food admission, further underscores the significance of adjusting dietary decisions to circadian rhythms. The body's circadian musicality impacts supplement digestion and energy use more than a 24-hour cycle. Customized nourishment plans might consider a person's circadian mood to streamline the planning of feasts, possibly working on metabolic wellbeing and supporting weight guideline.

Regardless of the promising capability of customized nourishment, challenges and moral contemplations should be tended to. Security concerns connected with hereditary information, the exactness of hereditary testing, and the potential for criticism in light of hereditary inclinations are significant perspectives to consider. Besides, the interpretation of logical discoveries into significant and down to earth dietary proposals requires continuous examination and approval.

The incorporation of customized sustenance into standard medical care brings up issues about availability and moderateness.

While hereditary testing has become more open, there are variations in admittance to medical care assets that might restrict the far and wide reception of customized sustenance draws near. Guaranteeing that the advantages of customized nourishment are accessible to different populaces is vital for address wellbeing disparities.

In the domain of general wellbeing, customized sustenance can possibly alter nourishment approaches and mediations. Getting away from conventional dietary rules could prompt more designated and viable techniques for forestalling diet-related illnesses. Legislatures and wellbeing associations might have to adjust their ways to deal with nourishment training and general wellbeing efforts to integrate customized sustenance standards.

Teaching medical care experts about customized sustenance is one more basic part of its incorporation into medical care frameworks. Doctors, dietitians, and other medical services suppliers should be furnished with the information and apparatuses to decipher and apply customized nourishment data in clinical settings. Proficient improvement programs and instructive assets can assume a vital part in planning medical services experts for the time of customized medication.

In the buyer domain, the prominence of customized sustenance is obvious in the ascent of direct-to-shopper hereditary testing administrations and customized feast arranging applications. These devices enable people to assume command over their wellbeing by giving customized experiences and suggestions. Nonetheless, the precision and unwavering quality of these administrations change, and customers ought to move toward them with a basic eye. Also, the understanding of hereditary data might require direction from medical services experts to guarantee informed navigation.

Social and dietary variety add one more layer of intricacy to the execution of customized nourishment on a worldwide scale. Various populaces have unmistakable dietary propensities, inclinations, and hereditary varieties. Altering sustenance proposals to suit different social settings is essential to guarantee the significance and viability of customized nourishment procedures around the world.

Chapter 8

Overcoming Challenges and Barriers

Defeating difficulties and obstructions is an inborn piece of the human experience. Over the entire course of time, people and social orders have confronted different impediments that have tried their versatility, assurance, and imagination. These difficulties can appear in various structures, going from individual battles to cultural issues, and they frequently require imaginative arrangements and an unflinching obligation to advance.

On an individual level, people experience a bunch of difficulties that shape their personality and characterize their life process. One normal deterrent is the quest for schooling and expert achievement. Many individuals face monetary imperatives, restricted admittance to quality instruction, or cultural assumptions that impede their scholar and profession goals. Regardless of these difficulties, people frequently track down ways of defeating such boundaries through difficult work, tirelessness, and a steady quest for their objectives.

Physical and emotional wellness moves likewise present huge hindrances to people taking a stab at a satisfying life. Persistent ailments, handicaps, and psychological wellness issues can affect one's capacity to connect completely in day to day exercises and seek after private objectives. Exploring these impediments requires clinical mediation as well as areas of strength for a framework, versatility, and a positive mentality. Numerous people have shown extraordinary strength in conquering wellbeing related difficulties, rousing others to confront their afflictions with boldness and assurance.

In the domain of connections, relational difficulties and boundaries can strain associations with family, companions, and significant others. Correspondence breakdowns, false impressions, and contrasts in values or viewpoints can make jumps that appear to be impossible. Constructing and keeping up with solid connections require compelling correspondence, compassion, and an eagerness to think twice about. Defeating these relational difficulties frequently includes self-awareness, self-reflection, and a guarantee to understanding and regarding others.

Cultural hindrances present considerable difficulties on a more extensive scale, influencing whole networks and populaces. Segregation, disparity, and unfairness can block progress and cutoff open doors for specific gatherings.

Accomplishing social change and destroying foundational obstructions require aggregate activity, support, and a pledge to equity. Since the beginning of time, different developments and people have battled against cultural treacheries, starting positive changes and preparing for an additional comprehensive and fair future.

Monetary difficulties likewise assume a huge part in molding the open doors accessible to people and networks. Destitution, joblessness, and monetary unsteadiness make hindrances to training, medical services, and generally prosperity. Defeating these monetary difficulties includes resolving foundational issues, advancing financial strengthening, and cultivating arrangements that advance equivalent open doors for all.

In the domain of innovation, the fast speed of headway can set out both open doors and difficulties. The computerized partition, where certain populaces need admittance to innovation and the web, represents a hindrance to data and open doors. Overcoming this issue requires drives zeroed in on computerized education, framework advancement, and guaranteeing fair admittance to innovation. Besides, moral contemplations and the likely abuse of innovation likewise present difficulties that require smart guideline and mindful advancement.

Ecological difficulties, for example, environmental change and cataclysmic events, present existential dangers to the planet and its occupants. Defeating these difficulties requests worldwide collaboration, feasible practices, and a promise to natural stewardship. The effect of environmental change is now obvious, with rising ocean levels, outrageous climate occasions, and loss of biodiversity. Addressing these difficulties requires aggregate endeavors to decrease fossil fuel byproducts, progress to environmentally friendly power sources, and execute economical practices across businesses.

Political difficulties, both homegrown and global, present complex obstructions to accomplishing harmony, dependability, and equity. Philosophical contrasts, epic showdowns, and international pressures can prompt struggle and upset progress. Defeating these political boundaries requires strategic endeavors, worldwide coordinated effort, and a pledge to maintaining basic liberties. History is loaded with instances of countries meeting up to conquer political difficulties, exhibiting the potential for positive change through discourse and collaboration.

Notwithstanding these diverse difficulties, people and social orders frequently draw on a scope of systems to defeat hindrances and cultivate positive change. Instruction arises as a useful asset for individual and cultural headway, outfitting people with the information and abilities expected to explore complex difficulties. Drives that elevate equivalent admittance to schooling, especially for underestimated networks, add to breaking the pattern of neediness and imbalance.

Development and innovation assume a vital part in beating boundaries by giving new answers for longstanding issues. Mechanical progressions in fields like medical care, farming, and correspondence can possibly further develop lives and set out open doors. Embracing advancement requires a pledge to innovative work, as well as strategies that support the mindful and moral utilization of innovation.

Social developments and support endeavors have generally assumed a vital part in beating cultural difficulties. Developments for social liberties, orientation uniformity, and ecological equity have ignited massive change by bringing issues to light, assembling networks, and pushing for strategy changes. Grassroots drives and local area drove endeavors frequently demonstrate successful in tending to nearby difficulties and advancing inclusivity.

Compelling authority is one more basic figure defeating difficulties, whether on an individual, local area, or worldwide level. Pioneers who have vision, compassion, and the capacity to rouse others can energize support for positive change. Initiative that focuses on cooperation, inclusivity, and long haul manageability is fundamental for exploring complex difficulties and encouraging strength inside networks.

Versatility, the capacity to return quickly from misfortune, is an ongoing idea among the individuals who effectively conquer difficulties. Versatile people and networks exhibit an ability to adjust to change, gain from misfortunes, and drive forward even with difficulty. Building flexibility includes developing a development mentality, creating survival strategies, and cultivating a steady climate that urges people to quickly return more grounded subsequent to confronting difficulties.

Social and cultural moves likewise add to conquering obstructions, as mentalities and standards develop over the long haul. Expanding mindfulness and comprehension of different viewpoints, encounters, and characters cultivates inclusivity and diminishes bias. Social moves that advance sympathy, resilience, and acknowledgment add to separating obstructions and making an additional agreeable and interconnected world.

Worldwide coordinated effort is fundamental in tending to worldwide difficulties that rise above public lines. Issues, for example, environmental change, pandemics, and helpful emergencies require facilitated endeavors from countries all over the planet. Associations like the Unified Countries assume a pivotal part in working with exchange, collaboration, and aggregate activity to address shared difficulties and advance worldwide harmony and thriving.

While beating difficulties is a general human encounter, the way to progress isn't direct or clear 100% of the time. Difficulties, disappointments, and snapshots of uncertainty are inescapable, however they likewise present open doors for development and learning. Embracing a mentality of constant improvement and review difficulties as venturing stones to progress can engage people and networks to explore obstructions with strength and assurance.

Taking everything into account, defeating difficulties and boundaries is a necessary piece of the human experience, forming people, networks, and social orders. From individual battles to worldwide issues, the excursion to beating hindrances includes a mix of training, development, backing, initiative, versatility, social movements, and global cooperation. By tending to difficulties at different levels and drawing on assorted systems, humankind can possibly construct a more evenhanded, reasonable, and comprehensive future. The accounts of the people who have defeated affliction act as motivation, helping us to remember the aggregate strength and versatility that can drive positive change even with difficulties.

8.1 Addressing common obstacles to maintaining a healthy diet.

Keeping a solid eating routine is an objective that numerous people try to accomplish, perceiving the critical effect that nourishment has on generally speaking prosperity. Nonetheless, in spite of the best goals, various normal snags frequently hold up traffic of sticking to a nutritious and adjusted eating plan. From occupied ways of life and restricted assets to mental variables and cultural impacts, tending to these difficulties is fundamental for advancing long haul wellbeing and forestalling the improvement of diet-related medical problems.

One common impediment to keeping a sound eating routine is the quick moving nature of current life. The requests of work, family, and different obligations can prompt feverish timetables that allow for insightful dinner arranging and arrangement. In the hurry to comply with time constraints and take care of different responsibilities, people might end up picking helpful however frequently less nutritious food decisions, like cheap food or pre-bundled dinners. Conquering this impediment requires a proactive way to deal with using time productively and a promise to focusing on wellbeing in the midst of the tensions of a bustling way of life.

Restricted admittance to new and reasonable produce is one more typical hindrance to taking on a solid eating regimen, especially for people dwelling in food deserts — regions where admittance to nutritious food is scant. In such conditions, the predominance of corner shops and cheap food outlets might eclipse the accessibility of new natural products, vegetables, and entire grains. Addressing this impediment includes pushing for further developed admittance to reasonable, top notch food in underserved networks, as well as supporting nearby drives that advance manageable horticulture and local area gardens.

Monetary requirements can likewise represent a huge test to keeping a sound eating regimen. Supplement thick food sources, for example, new produce and lean proteins, frequently accompany a greater cost tag contrasted with handled and less nutritious other options. This monetary obstruction might drive people and families to settle on splits the difference in their food decisions, possibly forfeiting nourishing quality for reasonableness. Carrying out approaches that make good food more open and reasonable, alongside elevating monetary proficiency to assist people with pursuing informed decisions, can add to defeating this snag.

Mental elements assume a critical part in dietary decisions, and profound eating is a pervasive hindrance for some people. Stress, fatigue, misery, and different feelings can set off a longing for solace food varieties that are much of the time high in sugar, salt, and undesirable fats. Breaking the pattern of close to home eating requires creating sound survival techniques, like care, exercise, or looking for help from loved ones. Moreover, cultivating a positive relationship with food through careful eating practices can add to a better way to deal with sustenance.

Social and social impacts likewise assume a huge part in molding dietary propensities. Family customs, social standards, and get-togethers frequently rotate around unambiguous food sources, which may not necessarily in all cases line up with a smart dieting plan. Offsetting social inclinations with dietary necessities includes tracking down imaginative ways of altering conventional recipes, investigating different cooking techniques, and taking part in open discussions with loved ones about the significance of wellbeing cognizant food decisions.

One more obstruction to keeping a solid eating routine is the predominance of misdirecting data in the media and on the web. The wealth of trend slims down, clashing nourishment exhortation, and sensationalized titles can make disarray and deception, making it moving for people to go with informed dietary decisions. Advancing sustenance training and media proficiency is fundamental in assisting individuals with exploring the immense measure of data accessible, empowering them to recognize proof based suggestions and unconfirmed cases.

Dietary limitations and food sensitivities add an additional layer of intricacy to the test of keeping a solid eating routine. People with explicit dietary necessities, like those following veggie lover or vegetarian ways of life, or those with gluten narrow mindedness, may confront trouble tracking down reasonable choices in different settings. Conquering this obstruction requires expanded mindfulness and convenience in food foundations, as well as enabling people with dietary limitations to advocate for their necessities and pursue informed decisions.

Instilled propensities and schedules, especially those created over numerous years, can be a considerable snag to taking on a better eating routine. Breaking liberated from the solace of recognizable yet undesirable eating designs requires a cognizant work to present progressive changes. Laying out new propensities, like integrating more leafy foods into feasts or picking entire grains over refined sugars, can add to long haul progress in keeping a sound eating routine.

The omnipresence of handled and comfort food sources in the cutting edge food scene presents one more test to those looking for a nutritious eating routine. These food sources, frequently high in sugar, salt, and unfortunate fats, are intended for accommodation and expanded time span of usability, however they might come up short on fundamental supplements required for ideal wellbeing. Conquering this snag includes a change in cultural standards and inclinations, advancing a culture that values entire, negligibly handled food varieties and focuses on nourishing substance over comfort.

Lacking sustenance training in schools and networks is a critical obstruction that adds to the propagation of unfortunate dietary propensities. Numerous people come up short on information about sustenance, segment sizes, and the significance of a decent eating regimen. Incorporating thorough sustenance instruction into school educational plans and local area projects can engage people to settle on informed decisions about their eating routine, encouraging a deep rooted obligation to wellbeing and prosperity.

Natural supportability is an undeniably perceived figure dietary decisions, and the ecological effect of food creation can impact choices about what to eat. A few people face the problem of picking either healthfully ideal choices and those that line up with their ecological qualities. Tending to this impediment includes advancing manageable cultivating works on, decreasing food squander, and empowering the utilization of plant-based food sources, which frequently have a lower ecological impression than creature items.

Changing socioeconomics and changes in family structures likewise add to difficulties in keeping a solid eating routine. Single-parent families, double pay families, and people living alone may find it trying to adjust work, providing care liabilities, and feast planning. Making steady local area programs, working environment strategies, and drives that work with admittance to nutritious, efficient dinners can assist people with exploring these difficulties and focus on their wellbeing.

The impact of showcasing and food promoting is an inescapable deterrent that can shape food decisions, particularly among kids and young people. The showcasing of unfortunate food sources, frequently high in sugar and low in healthy benefit, can add to the improvement of unfortunate dietary propensities since early on. Executing stricter guidelines on food publicizing to youngsters, advancing sustenance training in schools, and cultivating media proficiency can assist with balancing the adverse consequence of showcasing on dietary decisions.

Addressing the boundaries to keeping a solid eating routine requires a thorough and complex methodology that includes individual decisions, local area drives, strategy changes, and cultural mentalities toward food and sustenance. Enabling people with the information and abilities to pursue informed dietary decisions, elevating admittance to reasonable and nutritious food varieties, and establishing a climate that upholds solid propensities are vital parts of a fruitful technique.

Local area commitment and grassroots drives assume an imperative part in defeating snags to a sound eating regimen. Local area plants, ranchers' business sectors, and neighborhood nourishment projects can add to expanded admittance to new deliver and encourage a feeling of aggregate liability regarding wellbeing. Cooperation between neighborhood states, organizations, and local area associations is fundamental in establishing conditions that advance good food decisions and address the particular necessities of assorted populaces.

On a strategy level, there is a requirement for drives that advance food security, direct food publicizing, and backing manageable rural practices. Sponsorships for quality food varieties, limitations on promoting undesirable food sources to kids, and the execution of sustenance norms in schools are instances of strategy mediations that can add to defeating boundaries to a solid eating routine. Moreover, strategies that address food deserts and elevate evenhanded admittance to nutritious food can lastingly affect general wellbeing.

Working environment wellbeing programs likewise assume a urgent part in addressing snags to keeping a sound eating routine, perceiving the huge measure of time people spend at work. Businesses can carry out drives like nourishment training, admittance to solid bites, and adaptable planning for breaks to help workers in going with better decisions. Making a working environment culture that values worker prosperity adds to a positive climate that upholds sound way of life decisions.

8.2 Strategies for overcoming emotional eating, time constraints, and other challenges.

Techniques for beating difficulties like profound eating, time imperatives, and different boundaries to a sound way of life are fundamental for people endeavoring to further develop their general prosperity. These hindrances can fundamentally influence one's capacity to keep a sound eating routine, take part in standard active work, and oversee pressure successfully. By embracing designated techniques, people can foster strength, lay out better propensities, and explore the intricacies of present day life all the more effectively.

Profound eating, a typical test looked by numerous people, includes the utilization of food in light of feelings as opposed to hunger. Stress, fatigue, pity, and other profound states can set off the longing for solace food varieties, frequently high in sugar, salt, and undesirable fats. Defeating profound eating requires a multi-layered approach that tends to both the close to home and conduct parts of this test.

One powerful technique is creating care and mindfulness. Careful eating includes focusing on the tangible parts of food, like taste, surface, and smell, and monitoring appetite and totality signals. By developing care, people can break the programmed relationship among feelings and eating, considering more deliberate and controlled food decisions. Procedures like profound breathing, reflection, and journaling can likewise upgrade mindfulness and give elective survival strategies to dealing with feelings.

Laying out an emotionally supportive network is one more key procedure for defeating close to home eating. Offering sentiments and difficulties to companions, family, or a care group can offer close to home help and assist people with exploring troublesome minutes without depending on unfortunate eating designs.

Associating with other people who might be confronting comparable battles cultivates a feeling of local area and decreases sensations of detachment, building up the conviction that one isn't the only one in that frame of mind towards better propensities.

Distinguishing and tending to the main drivers of close to home eating is urgent for long haul achievement. Treatment or advising can be significant apparatuses for investigating hidden intense subject matters, creating ways of dealing with hardship or stress, and building flexibility. Understanding the profound triggers for gorging empowers people to execute designated mediations and supplant damaging things to do with better other options.

Dietary training and arranging assume a urgent part in conquering profound eating. Finding out about the dietary benefit of various food varieties and what they mean for in general wellbeing can engage people to settle on informed decisions. Making an even and fulfilling dinner plan, which incorporates different supplement thick food sources, diminishes the probability of going to comfort food sources in the midst of profound pain. Talking with an enrolled dietitian or nutritionist can give customized direction and backing in fostering a feasible and nutritious eating plan.

Time imperatives are an inescapable test that can obstruct people from embracing a sound way of life. Adjusting work, family obligations, and individual responsibilities frequently allows for feast arrangement, exercise, and taking care of oneself. Nonetheless, with vital preparation and prioritization, people can conquer time limitations and make wellbeing a focal concentration in their day to day routines.

One powerful system for overseeing time requirements is feast preparing. Investing committed energy every week arranging and planning dinners ahead of time can save important time during occupied work days. Cluster cooking and putting away divides in the fridge or cooler guarantee that sound, home-prepared feasts are promptly accessible, lessening the impulse to select cheap food or unfortunate accommodation choices.

Incorporating active work into a bustling timetable requires innovative preparation and a pledge to focusing on work out. Short, extreme focus exercises or integrating actual work into day to day schedules, like using the stairwell or strolling during breaks, can be effective methods for remaining dynamic when time is restricted. Also, planning ordinary activity meetings as non-debatable arrangements in one's schedule makes consistency and supports the significance of actual prosperity.

Time usage methodologies, like defining boundaries, designating undertakings, and staying away from lingering, add to better by and large productivity. Figuring out how to express no to unnecessary responsibilities and making a sensible timetable that considers both work and taking care of oneself forestalls burnout and cultivates a reasonable way of life. Time usage abilities are critical for making the important space to reliably participate in solid propensities.

Using innovation and mechanization can likewise be significant in conquering time imperatives. Feast arranging applications, wellness trackers, and online assets give helpful instruments to coordinating and overseeing wellbeing related exercises. Also, utilizing basic food item conveyance administrations, feast unit memberships, or employing help for family assignments can save time and lessen the pressure related with dealing with different obligations.

Adaptability and versatility are fundamental while tending to time limitations. Perceiving that timetables might change and surprising occasions might emerge permits people to change their arrangements without feeling overpowered. Embracing an outlook that values progress over flawlessness urges people to put forth constant attempts towards a better way of life, even notwithstanding time-related difficulties.

Monetary imperatives frequently cross with time requirements, making extra hindrances to a sound way of life. Restricted assets might lead people to settle on less expensive however less nutritious food choices or deter them from putting resources into wellness related exercises. Conquering monetary boundaries requires clever fixes and a guarantee to tracking down reasonable ways of focusing on wellbeing.

Financial plan well disposed dinner arranging is a functional methodology for tending to monetary requirements. Picking practical, supplement thick food sources, purchasing in mass, and exploiting deals and limits can assist with extending a spending plan while as yet focusing on nourishment. Arranging feasts around occasional and neighborhood produce can likewise add to cost investment funds and backing better dietary patterns.

Investigating reasonable activity choices is critical for defeating monetary obstructions to actual work. Strolling, running, and bodyweight practices require insignificant or no gear and should be possible at practically no expense. Numerous people group offer free or minimal expense wellness classes, and online stages give an abundance of assets to locally situated exercises that require negligible venture.

Local area assets and encouraging groups of people assume a crucial part in tending to monetary requirements. Food banks, local area nurseries, and neighborhood associations might offer help with admittance to nutritious food. Recreational areas, public venues, and philanthropic associations frequently give free or minimal expense amazing open doors for active work and health programs. Investigating these assets can assist people with defeating monetary boundaries and access the help they need for a better way of life.

Schooling and support are incredible assets for advancing fundamental change that tends to monetary requirements. Supporting approaches that further develop admittance to reasonable, nutritious food and upholding for expanded subsidizing for local area wellbeing drives add to establishing a climate where wellbeing is more available for everybody, paying little heed to monetary means.

Social impacts and cultural standards can influence people's decisions and ways of behaving connected with wellbeing. Beating these outside factors requires a blend of mindfulness, decisive reasoning, and purposeful endeavors to adjust individual qualities to wellbeing cognizant choices.

One viable system for exploring social impacts is taking on a socially delicate way to deal with wellbeing. Perceiving and regarding social customs and inclinations while as yet focusing on wellbeing permits people to work out some kind of harmony among legacy and prosperity. Tracking down ways of changing customary recipes to make them better, investigating different cooking techniques, and incorporating nutritious fixings into social dishes add to an all encompassing way to deal with wellbeing that respects social characters.

Open correspondence with loved ones about wellbeing objectives and way of life changes is pivotal in defeating social boundaries. Sharing the significance of a solid way of life and looking for help from friends and family establishes a strong climate that lines up with individual qualities. By including loved ones in the excursion toward better wellbeing, people can fabricate an organization of consolation and understanding.

Social ability in medical care and wellbeing experts is fundamental for offering customized and successful help. Experts who get it and regard different social foundations can offer direction that is delicate to individual inclinations and values. Searching out medical services suppliers, nutritionists, and wellness specialists who embrace social skill upgrades the probability of getting guidance that lines up with individual social characters.

Media proficiency assumes a basic part in beating cultural impacts that might advance unfortunate ways of behaving. Perceiving and addressing ridiculous magnificence principles, trend eats less, and sensationalized wellbeing claims in the media permits people to go with informed decisions in view of proof and their own qualities. Schooling on media education engages people to channel through the commotion and spotlight on data that upholds their wellbeing objectives.

Pushing for comprehensive and different portrayals in the media adds to a more exact impression of the populace's variety. Empowering news sources to include an assortment of body types, nationalities, and social foundations advances an additional comprehensive story that upholds positive self-perception and different viewpoints on wellbeing. Supporting drives that challenge destructive generalizations and advance a reasonable and comprehensive depiction of wellbeing is fundamental for making cultural change.

The computerized age has achieved exceptional admittance to data, yet it has likewise led to difficulties connected with falsehood, ridiculous assumptions, and correlation culture.

Virtual entertainment stages, specifically, can impact people's impression of wellbeing and self-perception. Fostering a solid relationship with web-based entertainment includes cognizant utilization, decisive reasoning, and defining limits.

One procedure for defeating the adverse consequence of virtual entertainment is organizing a positive and steady web-based climate. Following records that advance body inspiration, emotional well-being mindfulness, and proof based wellbeing data makes a feed that lines up with sound qualities. Unfollowing accounts that add to negative mental self portrait or correlation culture permits people to control the substance they are presented to.

Adjusting screen time and genuine cooperations is fundamental for keeping a solid relationship with web-based entertainment. Setting explicit time limits, assigning without screen zones, and focusing on eye to eye collaborations add to a more adjusted way of life. Zeroing in on certifiable associations and encounters lessens the potential for adverse impacts from virtual entertainment to affect emotional well-being and prosperity.

Instructive projects and missions that advance media proficiency and emotional wellness mindfulness assume a fundamental part in conquering cultural impacts. Giving people the devices to fundamentally assess media messages, figure out the effect of web-based entertainment on emotional well-being, and construct flexibility against cultural tensions adds to a more educated and enabled populace.

Natural elements, including the accessibility of good food choices, admittance to places of refuge for active work, and openness to ecological poisons, can essentially influence people's capacity to keep a solid way of life. Tending to these natural difficulties requires a blend of individual activities, local area drives, and promotion for more extensive fundamental changes.

One viable technique for beating ecological hindrances is local area commitment. Partaking in or starting local area projects, for example, making local area gardens, sorting out neighborhood cleanups, or upholding for more secure strolling and trekking ways, adds to the advancement of conditions that help wellbeing. Local area based drives engage people to team up on arrangements that address their particular ecological difficulties.

Pushing for strategy changes that focus on ecological wellbeing is essential for making enduring effect. Supporting drives that further develop admittance to parks and sporting spaces, control the promoting and dispersion of undesirable food varieties, and address natural treacheries adds to a better climate for all. People can take part in backing endeavors by drawing in with neighborhood government, joining local area associations, and supporting arrangements that advance natural maintainability.

Establishing a home climate that upholds solid propensities is a fundamental individual system for defeating natural hindrances. Loading the kitchen with nutritious food varieties, assigning a space for active work, and limiting openness to ecological poisons add to a home climate that lines up with wellbeing objectives. Going with purposeful decisions in the home climate supports sound ways of behaving and diminishes dependence on outside factors.

Transportation hindrances can likewise affect admittance to quality food and open doors for actual work. People confronting difficulties connected with transportation can investigate elective modes, like strolling, trekking, or utilizing public transportation. Upholding for further developed public transportation framework and making walkable networks adds to defeating transportation hindrances and advancing a more dynamic way of life.

Ecological supportability is an undeniably significant thought in wellbeing related choices. People can add to natural prosperity by pursuing eco-accommodating decisions, for example, lessening food squander, picking reasonable and privately obtained food varieties, and limiting single-use plastics. Way of life decisions that line up with natural supportability benefit both individual wellbeing and the soundness of the planet.

The assembled climate, including the format and plan of neighborhoods and work environments, altogether impacts active work levels. People can defeat natural boundaries by picking dynamic transportation choices, like strolling or trekking, whenever the situation allows. Upholding for metropolitan arranging that focuses on walkability, bicycle framework, and the making of green spaces adds to the advancement of conditions that help actual work.

Defeating natural hindrances requires an aggregate exertion that tends to both individual decisions and more extensive foundational changes. By upholding for arrangements that advance ecological wellbeing, partaking in local area drives, and pursuing economical decisions in day to day existence, people can add to establishing conditions that help better ways of life for them and people in the future.

All in all, conquering difficulties connected with close to home eating, time imperatives, social impacts, cultural standards, and ecological elements requires a complex and customized approach. People can foster versatility, cultivate better propensities, and explore outer difficulties by embracing procedures that address the particular hindrances they face. From developing care and building encouraging groups of people to pushing for strategy changes and advancing ecological manageability, people have the ability to defeat hindrances and make a way towards a better and seriously satisfying life.

8.3 Tips for building a supportive environment for nutritional success.

Establishing a steady climate is principal to making nourishing progress and cultivating long haul wellbeing and prosperity. The spaces wherein people live, work, and mingle essentially impact their dietary decisions, propensities, and generally way of life. Executing useful ways to fabricate a steady climate can enable people to pursue better decisions, lay out manageable propensities, and defeat normal hindrances to ideal sustenance.

1. **Home Climate:**

   Start by developing a supporting home climate. Stock the kitchen with different entire, supplement thick food sources, making it simple to get ready adjusted feasts. Sort out the storage room and cooler to focus on better choices, putting natural products, vegetables, and entire grains inside simple reach. Keep undesirable tidbits far away to decrease allurement, and consider distributing snacks ahead of time for better part control.

Feast readiness can be rearranged by arranging and preparing fixings quite a bit early. Put away unambiguous days for feast arranging, shopping for food, and clump cooking. Planning feasts in mass considers simple admittance to sound choices consistently, limiting the dependence on accommodation or quick food sources.

Energize family contribution in dinner arranging and planning. Drawing in youngsters in the kitchen gives significant fundamental abilities as well as cultivates an appreciation for nutritious food sources. Make a positive and charming climate during dinners by laying out standard family eating times, where everybody can share and interface over food.

2. **Careful Eating Practices:**

   Integrate careful eating rehearses into day to day schedules. Empower the propensity for plunking down to eat without interruptions, like TV or electronic gadgets. Focusing on yearning and totality signals advances a better relationship with food and forestalls gorging.

   Bite food gradually and enjoy each chomp to upgrade the eating experience and permit time for satiety signs to arrive at the cerebrum. Careful eating includes being available at the time, appreciating the flavors and surfaces of food, and perceiving the body's signals for yearning and fulfillment.

3. **Strong Social Associations:**

   Construct an organization of steady friendly associations with support positive dietary propensities. Share wellbeing objectives with loved ones, cultivating a climate where everybody urges each other to pursue nutritious decisions. Participate in exercises that advance prosperity, like cooking together, attempting new recipes, or partaking in proactive tasks collectively.

   Joining clubs or gatherings with an emphasis on wellbeing and sustenance can offer extra help and inspiration. Whether it's a nearby cooking club, wellness class, or online local area, interfacing with similar people makes a feeling of responsibility and shared obligation to healthful achievement.

4. **Work environment Wellbeing:**

   Advance work environment wellbeing by upholding for good dieting choices and drives. Urge bosses to give nutritious snacks in like manner regions, support wellbeing programs, and arrange occasions that underscore wellbeing and prosperity. Consider framing working environment wellbeing councils to start and support positive changes inside the association.

   Bring solid snacks and snacks to attempt to abstain from depending on candy machines or inexpensive food choices. Laying out an everyday practice for standard breaks, including short strolls or extending works out, adds to both physical and mental prosperity during the typical working day.

5. **Availability of Quality Food sources:**
Guarantee the availability of quality food sources in the neighborhood local area. Advocate for supermarkets to offer an assortment of new produce, entire grains, and lean proteins. Support neighborhood ranchers' business sectors or local area upheld farming (CSA) projects to get to new, privately obtained fixings.

Make people group cultivates or take part in existing ones to elevate admittance to new deliver and take part in feasible, neighborhood farming. Team up with nearby organizations and policymakers to address food deserts — regions with restricted admittance to reasonable and nutritious food — by executing arrangements like versatile business sectors or local area food drives.

6. **Sustenance Instruction:**
Focus on sustenance instruction inside the local area. Support drives that give studios, courses, or classes on nourishment and solid cooking. Training engages people with the information and abilities expected to pursue informed decisions about their eating routine.

Schools assume a basic part in sustenance training. Advocate for exhaustive sustenance educational programs that show kids the significance of adjusted feasts, food arrangement, and the effect of nourishment on in general wellbeing. Support approaches that work on the nature of school dinners and advance dietary mindfulness among understudies.

7. **Positive Food Informing:**
Be aware of the messages encompassing food decisions. Support positive language and perspectives towards food inside the family and local area. Try not to mark food varieties as "great" or "terrible" and center around advancing a reasonable and changed diet. Shift the account around food to one that underscores sustenance, satisfaction, and generally prosperity.

Support organizations and news sources that advance positive food informing and reject destructive eating regimen culture. Support the portrayal of assorted body types and dietary inclinations in promoting and media to encourage inclusivity and challenge unreasonable excellence guidelines.

8. **Active work Combination:**
Coordinate actual work into day to day schedules to supplement wholesome endeavors. Make spaces that support development, like home exercise regions or assigned outside spaces for work out. Consider integrating strolling or trekking into transportation techniques when possible.

Advance proactive tasks that line up with individual inclinations and interests. Whether it's moving, climbing, or partaking in group activities, tracking down agreeable ways of remaining dynamic improves generally speaking prosperity and supports dietary achievement. Laying out standard work-out schedules adds to a comprehensive way to deal with wellbeing.

9. **Innovation for Wellbeing:**

   Influence innovation to help dietary objectives. Use dinner arranging applications, nourishment trackers, and online assets for recipe thoughts. These instruments can improve on the most common way of overseeing dietary decisions, following supplement consumption, and remaining coordinated with feast arrangement.

   Investigate online wellness classes or virtual wellbeing networks for extra help and direction. Innovation offers an abundance of assets that take special care of individual inclinations and ways of life, making it simpler to coordinate wellbeing centered rehearses into day to day schedules.

10. **Objective Setting and Following Advancement:**

    Put forth clear and attainable dietary objectives to give guidance and inspiration. Characterize explicit, quantifiable, and sensible targets, whether they connect with consolidating more leafy foods, diminishing added sugars, or remaining hydrated. Consistently return to and change objectives to reflect changing needs and progress.

    Following advancement, whether through journaling, applications, or different techniques, upgrades responsibility and gives a substantial record of accomplishments. Celebrate achievements, regardless of how little, to support positive ways of behaving and keep up with inspiration on the excursion toward nourishing achievement.

11. **Culinary Abilities Advancement:**

    Focus profoundly on creating culinary abilities to upgrade the satisfaction in nutritious dinners. Go to cooking classes, try different things with new recipes, and investigate different cooking procedures. Building trust in the kitchen improves the probability of getting ready healthy and tasty dinners at home.

    Include relatives in cooking exercises to make a cooperative and charming experience. Showing kids essential cooking abilities since the beginning lays out an establishment for a deep rooted enthusiasm for planning and getting a charge out of nutritious food varieties.

12. **Practical Decisions:**

Think about the ecological effect of food decisions. Support feasible and privately obtained choices whenever the situation allows. Lessen food squander by arranging feasts, using extras innovatively, and treating the soil natural waste. These eco-accommodating practices add to both individual wellbeing and natural maintainability.

Advocate for organizations and policymakers to embrace feasible practices, like lessening single-use plastics and carrying out naturally cognizant bundling. By supporting manageability drives, people add to a better planet and advance moral and capable food creation.

All in all, fabricating a steady climate for dietary achievement includes a mix of individual decisions, local area drives, and backing for more extensive foundational changes. Establishing a home climate that focuses on nutritious choices, encouraging steady friendly associations, advancing work environment wellbeing, and upholding for open good food varieties locally are basic parts of a thorough way to deal with wellbeing.

Schooling, both at the individual and local area levels, assumes an essential part in enabling people with the information and abilities expected to pursue informed decisions about their eating regimen. Positive food informing, combined with a shift towards comprehensive portrayals in media, adds to a social climate that values wellbeing over hurtful excellence norms.

Coordinating innovation, defining sensible objectives, and following advancement upgrade individual responsibility and inspiration. Culinary abilities improvement and an emphasis on practical decisions further enhance the nourishing excursion, making it more charming and lined up with long haul prosperity.

At last, by executing these viable tips and cultivating a steady climate, people can make the circumstances important for dietary achievement. This approach goes past individual activities, stretching out to local area commitment and support for arrangements that advance wellbeing and prosperity for all.

Chapter 9

Sustaining Nutritional Wisdom for a Lifetime

Supporting healthful insight for a lifetime is a diverse undertaking that includes grasping the complexities of food, taking on careful dietary patterns, and embracing an all encompassing way to deal with generally prosperity. In our current reality where dietary patterns go back and forth, and nourishing data can be overpowering, laying out a groundwork of information that endures for the long haul is vital.

At the center of supporting healthful insight is the acknowledgment that food isn't simply fuel; it is a wellspring of sustenance for the body, psyche, and soul. The excursion towards supporting wholesome insight starts with developing a consciousness of the effect that food decisions can have on individual wellbeing and the more extensive climate. This mindfulness lays the foundation for going with informed choices that add to long haul prosperity.

One critical part of supporting dietary insight is grasping the idea of supplement thickness. Supplement thick food varieties give a high grouping of fundamental nutrients, minerals, and other helpful mixtures comparative with their calorie content. Focusing on supplement thick choices guarantees that each nibble adds to meeting the body's dietary requirements, advancing ideal wellbeing over the long haul.

Notwithstanding supplement thickness, the significance of a fair eating routine couldn't possibly be more significant. A balanced eating plan incorporates an assortment of nutritional categories, including organic products, vegetables, entire grains, lean proteins, and solid fats. This variety guarantees that the body gets a range of supplements, supporting different physiological capabilities and advancing by and large essentialness.

As people explore the complicated scene of dietary decisions, being knowing consumers is fundamental. Perusing food marks, understanding part estimates, and being aware of stowed away added substances enable people to pursue decisions lined up with their wellbeing objectives. The capacity to translate nourishing data furnishes people with the devices expected to explore the frequently befuddling universe of bundled food sources and pursue decisions that line up with their wellbeing and health targets.

In addition, supporting wholesome insight reaches out past individual wellbeing to envelop more extensive biological contemplations. Our decisions about the food we devour influence the climate, from rural practices to food transportation and waste. Embracing manageable and eco-accommodating eating rehearses contributes not exclusively to individual prosperity yet additionally to the soundness of the planet.

Developing nourishing insight likewise includes fostering a solid relationship with food. Careful eating, established in the act of being completely present during feasts, urges people to appreciate the flavors, surfaces, and fragrances of their food. This approach advances a more profound association with the demonstration of eating, cultivating a more noteworthy appreciation for the sustenance that food gives.

A basic part of supporting healthful insight is keeping up to date with progressing exploration and improvements in the field of sustenance. The logical comprehension of sustenance advances, and people focused on deep rooted prosperity ought to stay open to integrating new information into their dietary practices. Remaining informed enables people to adjust their dietary decisions in light of arising proof, guaranteeing that their way to deal with wellbeing remains proof based and successful.

As the excursion towards supporting wholesome insight unfurls, the job of actual work should not be ignored. Normal activity supplements a nutritious eating routine by supporting generally wellbeing, improving mind-set, and adding to weight the executives. The cooperative energy between smart dieting and active work makes a strong starting point for supported prosperity.

Chasing wholesome insight, it is likewise critical to perceive and address individual dietary necessities and limitations. Factors, for example, age, orientation, ailments, and social inclinations impact nourishing prerequisites. Fitting dietary decisions to individual necessities guarantees that nourishing objectives are met in a manner that is manageable and pleasant.

Feast arranging arises as an important device in the mission for supported healthful insight. Arranging dinners ahead of time permits people to go with smart decisions, stay away from latest possible moment unfortunate choices, and guarantee an equilibrium of supplements over the course of the day. Furthermore, dinner arranging can be an imaginative and pleasant cycle, cultivating a feeling of independence and fulfillment in one's dietary decisions.

In the steadily advancing scene of nourishment, the job of dietary examples and patterns can't be disregarded. From veggie lover and vegetarian ways of life to discontinuous fasting and ketogenic counts calories, people are given a bunch of choices. Supporting dietary insight includes basically assessing these patterns, taking into account individual necessities, and embracing approaches that line up with long haul wellbeing targets.

Moreover, the significance of hydration in keeping up with healthful equilibrium and by and large prosperity couldn't possibly be more significant. Water is fundamental for different physiological capabilities, including assimilation, supplement retention, and temperature guideline. Integrating a satisfactory admission of water into day to day propensities is an essential part of supporting healthful insight.

The social part of eating is another aspect that impacts healthful decisions. Imparting feasts to loved ones cultivates a feeling of association and local area, adding to generally speaking prosperity. Nonetheless, it is vital for work out some kind of harmony between friendly parts of eating and individual dietary objectives, guaranteeing that the common experience lines up with one's healthy benefits.

As people explore the intricacies of current life, stress the executives arises as an essential figure supporting nourishing insight. The connection among stress and dietary decisions is bidirectional - stress can impact food inclinations, and on the other hand, nourishment assumes a part in overseeing pressure. Taking on pressure decreasing practices, like care, reflection, and sufficient rest, supplements healthful decisions in advancing comprehensive prosperity.

With regards to supporting nourishing insight, the job of schooling couldn't possibly be more significant. Enabling people with the information and abilities to pursue informed dietary decisions lays the basis for a long period of wellbeing. Nourishment schooling ought to be open, proof based, and custom-made to different crowds, guaranteeing that people from varying backgrounds can profit from the insight of wholesome information.

The significance of cultivating dietary insight since the beginning can't be sufficiently underlined. Acquainting youngsters with various healthy food sources, instructing them about the dietary benefit of various fixings, and ingraining an affection for cooking make an establishment for a long period of sound propensities. By advancing wholesome proficiency in schools and networks, society can add to the prosperity of people in the future.

All in all, supporting dietary insight for a lifetime is a dynamic and diverse excursion that includes figuring out the standards of sustenance, pursuing careful food decisions, and embracing a comprehensive way to deal with prosperity. From supplement thickness and adjusted diets to supportable practices and careful eating, the mainstays of nourishing insight are interconnected and add to long haul wellbeing.

The excursion towards supported nourishing insight requires progressing learning, versatility, and a guarantee to individualized approaches. As people explore the intricacies of dietary patterns, ecological contemplations, and individual prosperity, they should remain receptive to their bodies, the more extensive local area, and the planet.

By developing a profound comprehension of the effect of food decisions, taking on careful eating practices, and embracing an all encompassing way to deal with prosperity, people can support wholesome insight for a lifetime. This excursion isn't an objective however a consistent course of development, transformation, and a guarantee to focusing on wellbeing in the entirety of its aspects. As we leave on this deep rooted mission for dietary insight, we prepare for a better, more supported, and versatile future.

9.1 Summarizing key takeaways from the book.

Summing up key focal points from the book on supporting wholesome insight for a lifetime is a chance to distil the fundamental standards and bits of knowledge that add to a comprehensive and informed way to deal with deep rooted prosperity. All through the pages, the book accentuates the significance of grasping food as more than simple food, perceiving its part in supporting the body, psyche, and soul. This basic viewpoint makes way for an excursion that incorporates supplement thickness, adjusted counts calories, maintainability, careful eating, knowing commercialization, and continuous training.

At the core of the book's message is the idea of supplement thickness. Supplement thick food sources, those plentiful in fundamental nutrients, minerals, and valuable mixtures comparative with their calorie content, structure the foundation of a well-being cognizant eating routine. Focusing on such food varieties guarantees that each nibble contributes definitively to meeting the body's healthful requirements. This approach upholds by and large wellbeing as well as gives a viable structure to supporting nourishing insight over a long period.

A vital part of supporting healthful insight is the accentuation on balance. A balanced eating routine that incorporates an assortment of nutrition classes — organic products, vegetables, entire grains, lean proteins, and solid fats — guarantees a wide range of supplements important for ideal wellbeing. This decent methodology perceives the collaboration between various food parts and their aggregate commitment to physiological capabilities.

Exploring the complicated scene of nourishing decisions requires an insightful outlook. The book highlights the significance of perusing food marks, understanding piece estimates, and being aware of stowed away added substances. This buyer mindfulness engages people to pursue informed choices lined up with their wellbeing objectives, encouraging a feeling of command over their dietary decisions.

Moreover, the book investigates the more extensive environmental effect of dietary choices. Manageable and eco-accommodating eating rehearses are situated as fundamental to individual prosperity and the soundness of the planet. By taking into account the natural ramifications of food decisions, people can add to a more manageable and agreeable relationship with the Earth.

Developing dietary insight likewise includes fostering a solid and careful relationship with food. The book advocates for careful eating, a training established in being completely present during dinners. This approach urges people to relish the tangible experience of eating, cultivating a more profound association with the sustenance that food gives. By dialing back and valuing the demonstration of eating, people can improve their general prosperity.

A continuous obligation to remaining informed is featured as a basic part of supporting healthful insight. Given the advancing idea of dietary science, the book urges people to keep up to date with examination and improvements in the field. This receptiveness to new data takes into account the variation of dietary practices in view of arising proof, guaranteeing that wholesome decisions remain proof based and powerful.

Actual work is perceived as a correlative part of an all encompassing way to deal with wellbeing. Ordinary activity upholds generally prosperity, improves temperament, and adds to weight the board. The cooperative energy between good dieting and active work makes a strong starting point for supported prosperity and builds up the interconnectedness of way of life factors.

Individualization is a common subject in the book, underscoring the significance of fitting dietary decisions to individual necessities, inclinations, and limitations. Factors, for example, age, orientation, ailments, and social contemplations impact healthful necessities. Perceiving and tending to these singular subtleties guarantees that wholesome objectives are met in a manner that is practical and pleasant.

The meaning of dinner arranging arises as a pragmatic device in the excursion towards supported wholesome insight. Arranging feasts ahead of time enables people to settle on smart decisions, stay away from hasty and possibly unfortunate choices, and guarantee a reasonable admission of supplements over the course of the day. Dinner arranging adds to wellbeing as well as be an imaginative and charming cycle, encouraging a feeling of independence in dietary decisions.

Dietary examples and patterns are investigated inside the setting of supported wholesome insight. From veggie lover and vegetarian ways of life to discontinuous fasting and ketogenic slims down, people are given a scope of choices. The book empowers a basic assessment of these patterns, considering individual requirements and taking on approaches that line up with long haul wellbeing goals.

Hydration arises as a basic mainstay of dietary insight. The book highlights the significance of a sufficient admission of water for different physiological capabilities, including processing, supplement ingestion, and temperature guideline. Integrating legitimate hydration into day to day propensities is underlined as a central component of supporting nourishing insight.

The social component of eating is recognized, featuring the job of shared feasts in cultivating a feeling of association and local area. While perceiving the worth of public eating encounters, the book urges people to offset social perspectives with their singular dietary objectives. This nuanced viewpoint guarantees that common dinners line up with one's healthy benefits.

Stress the executives is distinguished as a urgent consider supporting healthful insight. The equal connection among stress and dietary decisions is investigated, with the book upholding for pressure diminishing practices like care, reflection, and satisfactory rest. Overseeing pressure really supplements wholesome decisions, adding to all encompassing prosperity.

Schooling is situated as a foundation chasing supported healthful insight. Engaging people with information and abilities to pursue informed dietary decisions establishes the groundwork for a long period of wellbeing. The book advocates for available, proof based sustenance training that takes special care of assorted crowds, guaranteeing that people from different foundations can profit from the insight of nourishing information.

The significance of imparting healthful mindfulness since the beginning is underscored. Acquainting youngsters with various healthy food varieties, teaching them about dietary benefits, and cultivating an adoration for cooking make a strong starting point for a long period of sound propensities. The book battles that advancing wholesome proficiency in schools and networks adds to the prosperity of people in the future.

All in all, the book on supporting wholesome insight for a lifetime offers a far reaching and interconnected system for exploring the intricacies of dietary decisions. From supplement thickness and adjusted diets to maintainability, careful eating, and progressing schooling, the key important points stress a comprehensive way to deal with prosperity. By developing a comprehension of the effect of food decisions, taking on careful eating practices, and embracing a guarantee to individualized, proof based approaches, people can support wholesome insight all through their lives. This excursion is certainly not a static objective however a nonstop course of development, variation, and a commitment to focusing on wellbeing across physical, mental, and natural aspects. As people leave on this deep rooted journey for wholesome insight, they add to a better, more supported, and versatile future for them and the more extensive local area.

9.2 Providing a roadmap for integrating nutritional wisdom into a long-term, sustainable lifestyle.

Giving a guide to incorporating dietary insight into a long haul, practical way of life includes winding around together the different features of wellbeing and prosperity into a strong and versatile structure. As people endeavor to pursue educated and feeding decisions, this guide fills in as an aide, underlining the exchange between sustenance, way of life, and maintainability. It integrates standards like supplement thickness, adjusted slims down, care, schooling, and ecological cognizance to make an all encompassing methodology that can endure everyday hardship.

The excursion starts with a basic comprehension of supplement thickness. Supplement thick food varieties, those plentiful in fundamental nutrients, minerals, and gainful mixtures comparative with their calorie content, structure the bedrock of a wellbeing cognizant eating regimen. The guide urges people to focus on these food varieties, perceiving that they give the essential structure blocks to generally wellbeing and imperativeness. By embracing supplement thickness as a core value, people set up for supported nourishing insight.

Expanding upon the idea of supplement thickness is the significance of a reasonable eating regimen. A balanced eating plan that incorporates an assortment of nutrition types guarantees a different scope of supplements, adding to the ideal working of the body. The guide advocates for the incorporation of organic products, vegetables, entire grains, lean proteins, and solid fats, making an ensemble of supplements that upholds different physiological cycles. This equilibrium advances wellbeing as well as lays out a maintainable and versatile starting point for long haul prosperity.

Chasing nourishing insight, care arises as a vital component. The guide urges people to move toward eating with mindfulness, enjoying the flavors, surfaces, and smells of their food. Careful eating goes past the demonstration of devouring calories; it includes being completely present during feasts, encouraging a more profound association with the sustenance that food gives. By developing care, people can upgrade their relationship with food, settling on more deliberate and wellbeing advancing decisions.

A foundation of the guide is the idea of being an insightful customer. Exploring the advanced food scene requires the capacity to understand names, comprehend segment measures, and recognize stowed away added substances. The guide enables people to pursue informed decisions, perceiving that such insight is a critical part of supporting wholesome insight. By fostering the abilities to explore the intricacies of bundled food sources, people gain a feeling of command over their dietary choices.

Natural cognizance is entwined into the texture of the guide, perceiving that singular decisions influence the more extensive biological system. Manageable and eco-accommodating eating rehearses are featured as necessary to individual prosperity and the strength of the planet. The guide urges people to think about the natural impression of their food decisions, advancing an amicable connection between dietary choices and biological supportability.

Developing healthful insight includes a continuous obligation to training. The guide highlights the significance of remaining educated about advancements in the field regarding nourishment. Given the advancing idea of logical comprehension, people are urged to stay open to new data and change their dietary practices in light of arising proof. This flexibility guarantees that dietary decisions line up with the most recent logical bits of knowledge, adding to their viability and pertinence after some time.

Actual work is flawlessly coordinated into the guide as a corresponding component of an all encompassing way of life. Ordinary activity upholds in general wellbeing, upgrades temperament, and helps in weight the board. The collaboration between smart dieting and active work makes a hearty starting point for supported prosperity. The guide urges people to find exercises they appreciate, cultivating a positive relationship with development as a fundamental part of a solid way of life.

Personalization is a repetitive subject in the guide, perceiving that one size doesn't fit all in that frame of mind of sustenance. Individual factors, for example, age, orientation, ailments, and social inclinations impact healthful necessities. The guide urges people to tailor their dietary decisions to line up with their special conditions, guaranteeing that nourishing objectives are met in a manner that is reasonable and charming.

Feast arranging is introduced as a down to earth device inside the guide, offering an organized way to deal with pursuing deliberate and wellbeing cognizant food decisions. Arranging feasts ahead of time permits people to think about nourishing necessities, stay away from imprudent and possibly unfortunate choices, and guarantee a decent admission of supplements over the course of the day. Past its medical advantages, dinner arranging can be an imaginative and charming cycle, encouraging a feeling of independence in dietary decisions.

Dietary examples and patterns are tended to inside the guide, encouraging people to fundamentally assess famous methodologies and think about their reasonableness for long haul adherence. From veggie lover and vegetarian ways of life to discontinuous fasting and ketogenic slims down, the guide underscores the significance of adjusting dietary decisions to individual wellbeing targets. This insightful methodology guarantees that people take on supportable and sensible dietary examples that add to their general prosperity.

Hydration arises as a principal point of support inside the guide. Satisfactory water admission is perceived as fundamental for different physiological capabilities, including processing, supplement retention, and temperature guideline. The guide urges people to focus on hydration as a central part of their everyday daily schedule, perceiving its job in supporting by and large wellbeing.

The social component of eating is woven into the texture of the guide, recognizing the significance of shared dinners in encouraging associations and a feeling of local area. While perceiving the worth of mutual eating encounters, the guide underscores the requirement for people to figure out some kind of harmony between friendly angles and their singular dietary objectives. This nuanced viewpoint guarantees that common dinners line up with one's healthy benefits while adding to social prosperity.

Stress the board is coordinated into the guide as an essential part of supported healthful insight. The interchange among pressure and dietary decisions is investigated, with the guide supporting for pressure diminishing practices like care, contemplation, and satisfactory rest. By overseeing pressure successfully, people can establish a steady climate for settling on wellbeing advancing nourishing decisions.

Schooling is featured as a foundation inside the guide, underlining the significance of nourishing proficiency since the beginning. Imparting a comprehension of healthy food sources, dietary benefits, and the meaning of going with informed decisions lays the basis for a long period of wellbeing. The guide advocates for open, proof based sustenance schooling that takes care of assorted crowds, guaranteeing that people from different foundations can profit from the insight of nourishing information.

All in all, the guide for coordinating wholesome insight into a long haul, supportable way of life gives an extensive and interconnected guide for people looking to focus on wellbeing and prosperity. From supplement thickness and adjusted diets to care, schooling, and ecological cognizance, the critical components of the guide make a structure that is versatile, comprehensive, and persevering. As people set out on this excursion, they are enabled to pursue deliberate and wellbeing elevating decisions that add to their prosperity and the prosperity of the planet. The guide fills in as a compass, directing people towards a supportable and sustaining way of life that develops with the changing scene of nourishment and wellbeing.

9.3 Encouraging ongoing learning and adaptation as nutritional science evolves.

Empowering continuous learning and transformation as dietary science develops is an essential part of keeping a dynamic and informed way to deal with wellbeing and prosperity. In a quickly changing scene where new exploration discoveries consistently reshape how we might interpret nourishment, the significance of remaining educated and versatile couldn't possibly be more significant. This obligation to long lasting learning guarantees that people are outfitted with the most recent proof based data, permitting them to settle on informed dietary decisions that line up with their wellbeing objectives.

At the center of empowering progressing learning is a comprehension of the unique idea of wholesome science. The field persistently develops as scientists uncover new experiences into the connection among diet and wellbeing. Progressing studies investigate the effect of explicit supplements, dietary examples, and way of life factors on different parts of prosperity. By perceiving that nourishing science is a dynamic discipline, people can move toward their dietary decisions with a feeling of interest and receptiveness to new data.

One vital system for remaining informed is to draw in with legitimate wellsprings of healthful data. The expansion of data on the web expects people to be knowing purchasers, searching out proof based assets from solid sources.

Confided in wellbeing associations, peer-audited diaries, and qualified nourishment experts act as significant source for exact and state-of-the-art data. By developing a propensity for counseling definitive sources, people can filter through the tremendous ocean of wholesome data and pursue decisions established in logical proof.

The significance of decisive reasoning is underscored with regards to progressing learning. Not all nourishing data is made equivalent, and people should foster the abilities to perceive between sound logical proof and unsupported cases. The capacity to basically assess research studies, recognize connection and causation, and consider the more extensive setting of discoveries enables people to go with informed choices in view of the most ideal that anyone could hope to find proof. This basic outlook is a foundation of continuous learning in the domain of nourishment.

Embracing a development outlook is one more pivotal part of empowering continuous learning. A development mentality includes the conviction that one's capacities and knowledge can be created through devotion and difficult work. Applied to the setting of wholesome information, a development outlook urges people to see the excursion of finding out about sustenance as a continuous course of improvement and improvement. This viewpoint cultivates strength notwithstanding developing data and urges a proactive way to deal with remaining informed.

In the soul of progressing learning, people are urged to keep up to date with arising research discoveries. Logical examinations give significant experiences into the complicated associations among diet and wellbeing, and remaining informed about the most recent exploration permits people to as needs be adjust their dietary decisions. Buying into legitimate logical diaries, going to meetings, and following updates from wellbeing associations are procedures to remain associated with the front line of dietary science.

Be that as it may, moving toward new data with an insightful eye is fundamental. Single examinations, particularly those with little example sizes or restricted scope, may not give an exhaustive comprehension of a specific theme. Replication of discoveries and agreement inside established researchers add to the power of nourishing proof. Hence, people are urged to consider the heaviness of the general assemblage of proof as opposed to depending on separated examinations to illuminate their dietary choices.

As well as drawing in with logical writing, remaining associated with the more extensive nourishment local area is helpful for progressing learning. Partaking in gatherings, conversation gatherings, and networks zeroed in on nourishment permits people to share experiences, seek clarification on some pressing issues, and advantage from the aggregate information on a different gathering. Organizing with nourishment experts, teachers, and individual fans offers an important help framework for those exploring the intricacies of wholesome science.

Perceiving the singular idea of healthful necessities is a significant part of continuous learning and variation. While general dietary rules give an establishment to good dieting, individual varieties exist in view of variables, for example, age, orientation, medical issue, and individual inclinations. Understanding one's remarkable healthful necessities includes progressing self-reflection and a readiness to adjust dietary decisions in view of evolving conditions. Normal evaluations of wellbeing objectives, way of life changes, and developing nourishing necessities add to a customized and versatile way to deal with sustenance.

The job of innovation in working with continuous learning is featured inside the setting of nourishing science. Versatile applications, online stages, and wearable gadgets give instruments to people to follow their dietary propensities, screen wholesome admission, and get customized proposals. Utilizing innovation in this manner improves mindfulness and permits people to arrive at information informed conclusions about their sustenance. By embracing innovation as a partner chasing after wellbeing, people can incorporate continuous learning consistently into their regular routines.

Constant instruction about food marks is a fundamental piece of remaining informed and pursuing better decisions. Food bundling frequently contains an abundance of data, including wholesome realities, fixing records, and wellbeing claims. Understanding how to decipher this data engages people to settle on decisions lined up with their wellbeing objectives. Consistently refreshing information about naming guidelines and industry patterns guarantees that people can explore the supermarket with certainty, choosing food varieties that add to their prosperity.

As dietary science develops, the idea of bio-independence is stressed as a core value. Bio-distinction perceives that every individual is remarkable, and there is nobody size-fits-all way to deal with nourishment. Hereditary variables, microbiome creation, and metabolic contrasts add to individual varieties in how the body answers various food varieties. Embracing bio-distinction includes continuous self-disclosure, permitting people to distinguish the dietary examples that best help their special wellbeing and prosperity.

Empowering progressing advancing additionally includes cultivating wholesome education in the more extensive local area. Schooling drives pointed toward working on open comprehension of nourishment add to a more educated society. By supporting open and proof based nourishment training in schools, work environments, and networks, people can by and large add to a culture of wellbeing. Engaging others with the information and abilities to pursue informed dietary decisions makes a gradually expanding influence that broadens the advantages of progressing figuring out how to a more extensive crowd.

In the domain of continuous learning, the significance of culinary abilities is highlighted. Understanding how to plan nutritious and tasty feasts improves the common-sense utilization of wholesome information.

Cooking at home permits people to have more noteworthy command over the fixings in their feasts, explore different avenues regarding assorted flavors, and designer recipes to meet their healthful requirements. Continuous investigation of culinary methods and recipes adds to an economical and charming way to deal with smart dieting.

The guide for progressing learning in wholesome science reaches out past the domain of individual decisions to incorporate promotion for fundamental change. People are urged to draw in with and support drives that advance proof based nourishment arrangements. Taking part openly talk, supporting examination financing, and pushing for dietary training add to a cultural climate that focuses on wellbeing and prosperity. By effectively partaking in endeavors to shape the more extensive healthful scene, people assume a part in making a strong and informed local area.

All in all, uplifting continuous learning and transformation as wholesome science develops is a dynamic and proactive way to deal with wellbeing and prosperity. By perceiving the powerful idea of nourishing science, drawing in with legitimate sources, developing decisive reasoning, embracing a development outlook, and remaining associated with the sustenance local area, people can explore the intricacies of advancing data. The combination of innovation, nonstop training about food names, understanding bio-uniqueness, and encouraging wholesome proficiency add to a far reaching guide for progressing learning. As people set out on this excursion, they not just engage themselves with the information to pursue informed decisions yet in addition add to a culture of wellbeing and prosperity in the more extensive local area. In the steadily developing scene of wholesome science, the obligation to continuous learning guarantees that people are prepared to adjust their way to deal with sustenance in a manner that is proof based, feasible, and helpful for deep rooted prosperity.

The scene of nourishing science is dynamic and always showing signs of change, set apart by nonstop exploration, disclosures, and developing viewpoints. As how we might interpret the perplexing connection among diet and wellbeing extends, it becomes basic to energize progressing learning and variation. Exploring the developing landscape of nourishing science isn't simply a question of remaining current with the most recent discoveries; it is a comprehensive way to deal with deep rooted prosperity that includes decisive reasoning, receptiveness to new data, and a comprehension of individualized needs.

At the core of empowering continuous learning is the acknowledgment that healthful science is a dynamic field. New examinations, procedures, and experiences arise consistently, reshaping how we might interpret nourishment's job in wellbeing. It is pivotal for people to embrace an outlook that sees dietary information as liquid and dependent upon refinement. This viewpoint encourages a feeling of interest, provoking people to move toward wholesome data with a receptive outlook, prepared to adjust their dietary decisions in light of the latest proof.

Decisive reasoning is a foundation of exploring the developing scene of dietary science. With a wealth of data accessible through different channels, people should improve their skill to recognize between solid, proof based sources and possibly deceptive or one-sided claims. Figuring out the distinction among relationship and causation, assessing concentrate on systems, and taking into account the more extensive setting of exploration discoveries engages people to go with informed choices established in logical thoroughness.

Drawing in with trustworthy wellsprings of wholesome data is fundamental to remaining very much educated. Confided in wellbeing associations, peer-checked on diaries, and qualified nourishment experts act as solid source for proof based information. Developing the propensity for counseling definitive sources guarantees that people get precise and modern data, permitting them to arrive at informed conclusions about their dietary decisions.

A fundamental part of progressing learning is the obligation to keeping up to date with arising research discoveries. Logical examinations offer significant bits of knowledge into the perplexing associations between unambiguous supplements, dietary examples, and wellbeing results. Consistently captivating with the most recent examination permits people to adjust their dietary decisions in light of advancing proof. Buying into legitimate logical diaries, going to meetings, and following updates from wellbeing associations are powerful procedures for remaining associated with the front line of dietary science.

Nonetheless, the coordination of new data requires an insightful methodology. Only one out of every odd review holds equivalent weight, and separated discoveries may not give a thorough comprehension of a specific point. The dependability of examination discoveries is improved when there is agreement inside established researchers and when studies are reproduced. Hence, people are urged to consider the heaviness of the general collection of proof instead of depending on disengaged investigations to illuminate their dietary choices.

Embracing a development mentality is essential for people exploring the complex and advancing field of healthful science. A development outlook includes seeing the method involved with finding out about nourishment as a continuous excursion of advancement and improvement. It urges people to move toward difficulties with strength, perceiving that mishaps and developing data are essential pieces of the educational experience. This mentality cultivates a proactive demeanor toward remaining informed and adjusting dietary decisions in light of the most recent proof.

In the soul of progressing learning, people are urged to associate with the more extensive nourishment local area. Taking part in gatherings, conversation gatherings, and networks zeroed in on sustenance gives a stage to sharing experiences, seeking clarification on pressing issues, and profiting from the aggregate information on a different gathering. Organizing with nourishment experts, teachers, and individual devotees establishes a strong climate for those exploring the intricacies of wholesome science.

Remaining informed about healthful science includes perceiving the singular idea of nourishing necessities. While general nourishing rules give an establishment to good dieting, individual varieties exist in view of variables, for example, age, orientation, medical issue, and individual inclinations. Understanding one's novel healthful necessities includes progressing self-reflection and an eagerness to adjust dietary decisions in view of evolving conditions. Standard evaluations of wellbeing objectives, way of life changes, and developing nourishing necessities add to a customized and versatile way to deal with sustenance.

Innovation assumes a huge part in working with continuous learning in the domain of healthful science. Versatile applications, online stages, and wearable gadgets give apparatuses to people to follow their dietary propensities, screen healthful admission, and get customized proposals. Utilizing innovation upgrades mindfulness and permits people to come to information informed conclusions about their sustenance. By embracing innovation as a partner chasing after wellbeing, people can incorporate continuous learning flawlessly into their day to day routines.

Constant instruction about food names is a basic piece of remaining informed and settling on better decisions. Food bundling frequently contains an abundance of data, including nourishing realities, fixing records, and wellbeing claims. Understanding how to decipher this data engages people to settle on decisions lined up with their wellbeing objectives. Consistently refreshing information about marking guidelines and industry patterns guarantees that people can explore the supermarket with certainty, choosing food varieties that add to their prosperity.

Bio-uniqueness is a core value inside the continuous educational experience. Perceiving that every individual is remarkable, with particular hereditary variables, microbiome organization, and metabolic contrasts, underscores the requirement for an individualized way to deal with sustenance. Bio-singularity includes continuous self-disclosure, permitting people to recognize the dietary examples that best help their one of a kind wellbeing and prosperity. It energizes a customized and versatile way to deal with sustenance that perceives and regards individual varieties.

Empowering continuous advancing likewise includes encouraging healthful proficiency in the more extensive local area. Public comprehension of nourishment adds to a more educated society and enables people to settle on better decisions. Supporting open and proof based nourishment training in schools, work environments, and networks makes a culture of wellbeing. By effectively taking part in endeavors to advance nourishing proficiency, people add to a local area that values informed dynamic about food and sustenance.

Inside the domain of continuous learning, the significance of culinary abilities is highlighted. Understanding how to plan nutritious and delightful feasts upgrades the reasonable utilization of wholesome information.

Cooking at home permits people to have more prominent command over the fixings in their feasts, explore different avenues regarding assorted flavors, and designer recipes to meet their nourishing necessities. Progressing investigation of culinary strategies and recipes adds to a supportable and charming way to deal with good dieting.

Backing for fundamental change is introduced as an augmentation of continuous learning. People are urged to draw in with and support drives that advance proof based sustenance approaches. Partaking out in the open talk, supporting exploration subsidizing, and upholding for dietary schooling add to a cultural climate that focuses on wellbeing and prosperity. By effectively taking part in endeavors to shape the more extensive wholesome scene, people assume a part in making a steady and informed local area.

All in all, reassuring continuous learning and variation as wholesome science advances is a functioning and multi-layered way to deal with deep rooted prosperity. By perceiving the unique idea of wholesome science, drawing in with legitimate sources, developing decisive reasoning, embracing a development mentality, and remaining associated with the nourishment local area, people can explore the intricacies of developing data. The reconciliation of innovation, persistent instruction about food marks, understanding bio-independence, encouraging nourishing education, and embracing culinary abilities add to an extensive guide for continuous learning. As people leave on this excursion, they not just engage themselves with the information to settle on informed decisions yet in addition add to a culture of wellbeing and prosperity in the more extensive local area. In the steadily developing scene of wholesome science, the obligation to continuous learning guarantees that people are prepared to adjust their way to deal with nourishment in a manner that is proof based, supportable, and helpful for deep rooted prosperity.